T0173939

ANALYSING SOCIAL WORK COMMUNICATION

With communication and relationships at the core of social work, this book reveals the way it is foremost a practice that becomes reality in dialogue, illuminating some of the profession's key dilemmas. Applied discourse studies illustrate the importance of talk and interaction in the construction of everyday and institutional life.

This book provides a detailed review and illustration of the contribution of discourse approaches and studies on professional interaction to social work. Concentrating on how social workers carry out their work in everyday organisational encounters with service users and colleagues, each chapter uses case studies analysing real-life social work interactions to explore a concept that has relevance both in discursive studies and in social work. The book thus demonstrates what detailed discursive studies on interaction can add to professional social work theories and discussions. Chapters on categorisation, accountability, boundary work, narrative, advice-giving, resistance, delicacy and reported speech review the literature and discuss how the concept has been developed and how it can be applied to social work.

The book encourages professional reflection and the development of rigorous research methods, making it particularly appropriate for post-graduate and post-qualifying study in social work where participants are encouraged to examine their own professional practice. It is also essential reading for social work academics and researchers interested in language, communication and relationship-based work and in the study of professional practices more generally.

Christopher Hall is Social Care Researcher in the School of Medicine, Pharmacy and Health at Durham University, UK.

Kirsi Juhila is Professor in Social Work at the School of Social Sciences and Humanities at the University of Tampere, Finland.

Maureen Matarese is Assistant Professor in Developmental Skills at Borough of Manhattan Community College, CUNY, USA.

Carolus van Nijnatten is Professor in Social Studies of Child Welfare in the Faculty of Social and Behavioural Sciences at the University of Utrecht, Netherlands.

Routledge Advances in Social Work

New titles:

Analysing Social Work Communication
Discourse in practice
Edited by Christopher Hall, Kirsi Juhila, Maureen Matarese and Carolus van Nijnatten

Forthcoming titles:

Chronic Illness, Vulnerability and Social Work
Liz Walker and Elizabeth Price

Feminisms in Social Work Research
Edited by Stephanie Wahab, Ben Anderson-Nathe and Christina Gringeri

Social Work in a Global Context
Issues and challenges
Edited by George Palattiyil, Dina Sidhva and Mono Chakrabarti

ANALYSING SOCIAL WORK COMMUNICATION

Discourse in practice

Edited by Christopher Hall,
Kirsi Juhila, Maureen Matarese
and Carolus van Nijnatten

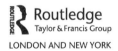

Routledge
Taylor & Francis Group

LONDON AND NEW YORK

First published 2014
by Routledge
2 Park Square, Milton Park, Abingdon, Oxon, OX14 4RN

Simultaneously published in the USA and Canada
by Routledge
711 Third Avenue, New York, NY 10017

Routledge is an imprint of the Taylor & Francis Group, an informa business

British Library Cataloguing in Publication Data
A catalogue record for this book is available from the British Library

Library of Congress Cataloging in Publication Data
Analysing social work communication: discourse in practice/
edited by Christopher Hall, Kirsi Juhila, Maureen Matarese and
Carolus van Nijnatten. – 1st Edition.
    pages cm. – (Routledge advances in social work)
    1. Social service.   2. Social interaction.   I. Hall, Christopher.
    HV40.A74223 2013
    361.301'4 – dc23
    2013013908

ISBN: 978-0-415-63682-7 (hbk)
ISBN: 978-0-415-71216-3 (pbk)
ISBN: 978-0-203-08496-0 (ebk)

Typeset in Sabon and Gill Sans
by Florence Production Ltd, Stoodleigh, Devon, UK

CONTENTS

CONTRIBUTORS

The contributors to this book are members of an international research group, *Discourse and Narrative Approaches to Social Work and Counselling* (DANASWAC). First established in 1997, the group has worked together on a number of research projects and has published widely on the subject. The contributors are from seven countries and most of the chapters are international collaborations.

Dorte Caswell is Associate Professor in social work in the Department of Sociology and Social Work at Aalborg University, Denmark.

Christopher Hall is Social Care Researcher in the School of Medicine, Pharmacy and Health at Durham University, UK.

Arja Jokinen is Senior Lecturer in social work at the School of Social Sciences and Humanities at the University of Tampere, Finland.

Kirsi Juhila is Professor in social work at the School of Social Sciences and Humanities at the University of Tampere, Finland.

Åsa Mäkitalo is Professor in Education in the Department of Communication, Education and Learning at the University of Gothenburg, Sweden.

Maureen Matarese is Assistant Professor in developmental skills at Borough of Manhattan Community College, CUNY, USA.

Martine Noordegraaf is Professor (lector) of youth and family and Lecturer of qualitative research methods at Christian University of Applied Sciences, Netherlands.

Suvi Raitakari is Researcher in social work at the School of Social Sciences and Humanities at the University of Tampere, Finland.

Sirpa Saario is Researcher in social work at the School of Social Sciences and Humanities at the University of Tampere, Finland.

Stef Slembrouck is Professor of English Linguistics and Head of the Linguistics Department at Ghent University, Belgium.

Eero Suoninen is Senior Lecturer in social psychology at the School of Social Sciences and Humanities at the University of Tampere, Finland.

Carolus van Nijnatten is Professor in social studies of child welfare in the Faculty of Social and Behavioural Sciences at the University of Utrecht, Netherlands.

ACKNOWLEDGEMENTS

We would like to thank the many colleagues who have supported, encouraged and challenged our discursive interaction studies during the last decade. The origin of the book was the sixth DANASWAC (*Discourse and Narrative Approaches to Social Work and Counselling*) meeting in Ghent (August, 2009), where we organised a round-table discussion dealing with different discursive approaches and their applicability in social work studies. Since then the book has been discussed and developed yearly in DANASWAC meetings. We wish to thank all the members of the DANASWAC network for valuable comments and inspiration. Some of the early versions of the chapters were also presented at the European Conference of Social Work Research in Oxford (March, 2011), where we arranged a symposium about discursive studies in social work.

Chapters 1, 2, 8 and 10 have been partially written based on findings from the research project *Responsibilization of Professionals and Service Users in Mental Health Practices*, led by Kirsi Juhila and funded by the Academy of Finland (2011–2016).

Chapter 3 was written within the *Linnaeus Centre for Research on Learning Interaction and Mediated Communication in Contemporary Society* (LinCS), a CoE financed by the Swedish Research Council (2006–cont.).

Chapters 5, 6 and 7 have drawn on data collected for the research projects *E-Assessment in Child Welfare*, led by Christopher Hall and funded by the Economic and Social Research Council e-Society programme (2005–2007), and *Error, Responsibility and Blame in Child Welfare*, led by Sue White (Birmingham University) and funded by the Economic and Social Research Council Public Services Programme (2007–2009).

The authors of Chapter 9 wish to thank Els Brouwer for helping with the data collection and for making verbatim texts. They also want to thank the Dutch Child Protection Board and its clients for their participation in the study.

1

SOCIAL WORK DISCOURSE
IN PRACTICE

Christopher Hall, Kirsi Juhila, Maureen Matarese
and Carolus van Nijnatten

Social work relies fundamentally on good communication, on empathetic
but purposeful talking and listening. In the process of developing supportive
relationships, communication with clients aims to gain information, identifying and assessing problems and making the right decisions. In order
to do this effectively and successfully social workers' communication skills
are crucial. These skills include, among other things, the ability to listen
carefully, to ask the right questions, to give clear advice and to pay attention
to all the relevant details in conversations with clients. Communication with
clients forms the basis for making judgements about what actions to take.
Hence, developing communication skills is one of the core goals in social
work education. In a recent review of teaching communication skills in social
work by the Social Care Institute for Excellence in the UK, communication
is seen as essential to social work:

> Learning to communicate in a professional manner in a variety of
> contexts with people from a diverse range of backgrounds can
> be difficult, but it is a fundamental skill without which it is difficult
> to perform many other social work tasks or, perhaps, the social work
> role at all.
>
> (Trevithick *et al.* 2004: 1)

Seeing good communication skills as an indispensable precondition
for good social work is a familiar idea in the social work field. It has been
written about extensively in professional social work literature, and various
textbooks and manuals contain lists of elements of good professional
communication and guidelines on how they can be achieved. This book also
addresses social work communication, but takes a different stance. It focuses

on the ways social workers carry out their work in everyday organisational conversations with clients and other professionals, and provides tools to analyse these conversations in great detail. This approach does so without determining in advance the characteristics of good or bad social work communication. The primary aim is not to offer recipes for good communication, but to make visible the richness and skilfulness of face-to-face interaction in real-life social work conversations. This means studying discourse in practice by utilising various discursive research approaches.

The discursive turn in social work research

Discourse studies have had a major impact across the social sciences over the last 40 years, illustrating the importance of talk and interaction in the construction of everyday life. Studies have concentrated on the ways in which social life is more than merely the outcome of personality or social structure. Instead, social encounters are seen as sites for creating social realities, as people manage a wide variety of negotiations, dilemmas and actions. Goffman (1983: 8) identifies the importance of studying 'the interaction order' of organisations:

> there is the obvious fact that a great deal of the work of organizations – decision-making, the transmission of information, the close coordination of physical tasks – is done face-to-face, requires being done in this way, and is vulnerable to face-to-face effects . . . there are people-processing encounters, encounters in which the 'impression' subjects make during the interaction affects their life chances.

The focus of investigation is on what actually happens in everyday talk and interaction, while recognising contextual constraints. The study of institutional interaction has been a particularly important topic for research, as doctors, therapists, teachers, public service workers or administrative staff manage encounters with service users, operating within organisational and professional expectations and role boundaries (e.g. Mchoul 1978; Silverman 1987; Atkinson 1995; Peräkylä 1995; Vehviläinen 1999; Mäkitalo 2002; Kurri 2005; Heritage and Maynard 2006; Peräkylä *et al.* 2008a). Rather surprisingly, social work has rarely been the focus of such studies, despite the centrality of talk and interaction to social work.

However, in the last decade, social work research and learning has also begun to utilise discursive methods. From this perspective, language and interaction play a dominant role, revealing that the way social work is implemented is primarily a practice that becomes established in dialogue. This type of research is especially relevant, as compared to many other professions, talk and interaction are the backbone of social work. This discursive turn in social work research follows developments in social science research and has led to increased study of everyday social interaction, utilising a variety of discourse methodologies and approaches.

Over the last ten years the number of studies of naturally occurring social work interaction has increased so that it can now be seen as a significant accumulation of knowledge (which we review and develop further in the following chapters). This development can be described as a change from analysis focusing on the contents of interaction (what kind of identities, problems etc. are constructed in interaction) towards analysis combining the detailed analysis of content and interactional devices present in social work encounters. It is an orientation towards not only *what* is said, but *how* it is said and the interaction between the two. Analysis that considers solely the content of data will see extracts of talk as representative of a topic, for example talk about foster care. In contrast, discourse analysis is interested in how talk is consequential for the management of a particular interaction. For example, how is talk about foster care introduced into a conversation to manage a decision to take a child into care? A distinction is made between 'topic' and 'resource' – how far is foster care the topic of the interaction or a resource to help manage the interaction.

Along with this development, research methodologies and methods have advanced considerably. These approaches have a number of advantages over traditional research methods. First, they examine actual interactions in social work settings, not participants' recollections of social work practice. Second, they are inductive, developing findings from data rather than seeking to confirm preformed hypotheses. Third, they concentrate on detailed and rigorous analysis and can be applied to small as well as larger data sets. Fourth, the display of actual encounters means that practitioners and service users can readily identify with the data examined and engage with the analysis.

Some approaches to social work have embraced 'evidence-based practice' in recent years, with the implication that only quantitative, quasi-experimental or randomised controlled trials count as appropriate evidence. Counter to this view, it has been argued that there are dangers in reducing the complexity of social work to simplistic procedures that apply statistical analysis to social work interventions, leading to rational decision making. Webb (2000) argues that social workers make decisions on the basis of 'a reflective deliberation process', not evidence. Discourse approaches to social work provide a wider range of contexts of social work practices, to expand and complicate what counts as both evidence and reflection.

Discursive and professional key concepts

This book aims to consolidate the development of discursive studies of social work talk and interaction. The purpose is not, however, to concentrate on research methods only. There are plenty of excellent textbooks available about different discursive approaches concentrating on talk and interaction (e.g. Antaki and Widdicombe 1998; Wood and Kroger 2000; Taylor and Wetherell 2001; Wetherell *et al.* 2001; Francis and Hester 2004; ten Have 2007; Silverman 2011) and on talk in institutional interaction (e.g. Drew and Heritage 1992b; Firth 1995; Gubrium and Holstein 2001). There is also some literature that focuses on institutional interaction in social work and related human service professions, for instance from the points of view of problem and client construction (e.g. Jokinen *et al.* 1999; Taylor and White 2000; Seltzer *et al.* 2001; Hall *et al.* 2003, 2006; Gubrium and Järvinen 2013). What is missing so far is a book that establishes links between professional social work discussions and theories and discursive interaction studies. This book will address this gap by providing a review of how the study of talk and interaction can illuminate some of the key dilemmas of social work.

We will do this by reviewing some of the main analytical concepts that have emerged from detailed discursive analyses of institutional encounters in different human service settings. For example, discourse studies illustrate how advice-giving is inevitably a feature of professional–service user meetings. Furthermore, it is a topic that must be handled carefully by participants since rejection of advice can cause interactional difficulties. Advice-giving is a familiar topic in the professional social work literature as well, but it is normally treated as a method to be deployed (or more often resisted) by a social worker when deciding on the intervention for a particular service user. Advice-giving is treated more like a skill of social workers without paying much attention to real-life encounters, where advice-giving is inevitably a feature of encounters in which social workers and clients meet, deployed to manage interactional expectations and obligations. The main idea is thus to demonstrate what detailed discursive studies on interaction can add to professional social work theories and discussions on certain familiar topics, to make 'seen but unnoticed' social work practices visible (Garfinkel 1967).

There are obviously many topics in social work that are a feature of everyday social work interaction that could be included in this book. The selection of concepts examined in the book is based, first, on a review of the available discursive interaction studies that address prevailing and timely discussions in professional social work literature and, second, on an assessment of what interaction studies – although often conducted in different human service settings – could add to these discussions. Hence, the concepts have relevance both in discursive studies and in social work. The concepts we selected for thorough examination are: categorisation, accountability, boundary work, narrative, advice-giving, resistance, delicacy and reported speech. The list is not complete in the sense that other concepts could have been considered for inclusion in the book, such as empathy, emotion and assessment. However, this selection of concepts covers many important topics and core discussions in social work.

When examining the key concepts our point of departure is that the comparisons across different settings are possible and useful. Comparisons are possible in three senses. First, social workers have much in common with other human service professionals, such as doctors, nurses, therapists, counsellors, educators and the police. All these professionals work near their patients or clients. They have conversations with them and conversation plays a crucial role in their work. Accordingly, discursive interaction research conducted in these different professional fields provides valuable insights also into social work studies and into the discursive and professional concepts examined in this book. Categorisation, giving accounts, doing boundary work, constructing narratives, giving advice, resisting, doing delicacy and using reported speech are all common interactional acts in social worker–client conversations as they are in other human service encounters. Second, the same holds true in different social work contexts and in work with different client groups. And, third, we also claim that similar interactional phenomena can be located in different countries' social work settings. This is not to say, however, that professional, organisational and country-specific contexts do not matter. They certainly matter and should be considered in doing interaction studies. Categorisation, doing delicacy, resisting and so on have similar features in all interaction, but when analysing them in different contexts with certain institutional goals they inevitably produce different contents, functions and consequences. For instance, clients' resistance to social workers' interpretations in voluntary occupational counselling sessions or in child protection meetings inevitably has different institutional functions and consequences. That is why institutional contexts ought to be taken carefully into account when doing interaction analysis and examining the display of key concepts in social work. However, everyday interaction and possible variations between different institutional settings and countries should not be explained 'top down'. Instead, the analysis starts from the micro level: how contexts are present and made sense of in interaction.

The data extracts examined in the chapters come from various social work contexts, including child protection and family work, services for substance abusers and for people suffering from mental health problems, community care for older people, domestic violence work, probation work, homeless people's shelters and job centres. The variety of institutional settings is thus rich. The richness applies also to countries the data are from: Finland, Denmark, England, the Netherlands, Sweden and the United States. As we stated above, the key concepts are not tied to certain kinds of social work, but are common in all social work interactions, although might have different characteristics in particular institutional settings and cultural contexts.

Naturally occurring data

As the focus of this book is on real-life, face-to-face social work interaction, the illustrative data we display in introducing and discussing the key concepts are 'naturally occurring'. This means that the data have been audio-recorded in authentic social work situations, such as social worker–client conversations, case conferences and team meetings among social workers. Hence, we do not use, for instance, interviews or focus group discussions arranged by researchers for the purposes of collecting research data.

The illustrative data have not been gathered for the purpose of this book. Some of the data extracts are borrowed from previously published studies, but the majority of them come from the authors' own studies. We all have long histories of conducting social work interaction studies and the data were collected in various research projects. Getting access to naturally occurring social work interaction is often a long and multistage process, starting from contacting key persons in institutions and then going through research ethical procedures. Such processes are discussed in textbooks on qualitative research methods (e.g. ten Have 2007; Silverman 2011). What is discussed less frequently is how to create trusting relations with participants in research settings before audio-recordings can commence. Despite a long tradition of research involving audio- and video-recording of patient–GP consultations, a recent literature review found that around 20 per cent of patients and 40 per cent of GPs refused to take part in this kind of research (Themessl–Huber *et al.* 2008). Social work has less of a tradition of being observed and recorded, as Pithouse (1998) points out: it is an 'invisible trade'. Our way to conduct research is ethnographic, which means that the researchers are present in the studied organisations, and they get to know people and institutional routines by observing practices and by discussing with managers, social workers and clients during the process of data gathering. We also often conduct interviews and collect institutional documents in order better to understand the settings. From our experience, getting access to often delicate interactional data is easier if the researchers are known and trusted in the organisations.

Research ethics is not only about getting official statements from ethical committees, receiving research permissions from social work organisations or collecting consent forms from individual people involved. It is first of all an issue of creating trusting relationships. This demands that social workers, clients and others involved are getting enough information about the research, they have real options to refuse their participation in research, their views of research are heard and taken into account, their voices in the recorded conversations are analysed respectfully, they are given possibilities to comment on research results and sometimes they are even invited to act as co-analysers of research data. In our own research projects we have tried to follow these kinds of ethical principles. Ethical questions are the subject of books on research methods (e.g. D'Cruz and Jones 2004) and papers in journals such as *Qualitative Social Work* and *Ethics and Social Welfare*.

When the research is concerned with the details of social work interaction, it is necessary to transcribe data carefully. This includes sometimes marking the pauses, loud and quiet talk, overlapping talk and so on, in addition to word by word verbal transcribing. The detail of transcriptions varies between the chapters, depending on the key concept in question. Transcription symbols are presented in the Appendix on page 181. Obviously, all the data extracts have been anonymised. Since our data come from different countries, the original languages include English, Finnish, Danish, Dutch and Swedish. This means that many extracts have been translated from another language to English. Translating everyday talk is a challenging, and never straight-forward process. Languages can carry meanings that are sometimes almost impossible to translate directly. However, translating is inevitable if we wish to discuss and compare data across countries and language areas. In trans-lations we have aimed to be as loyal to the original expressions as possible without losing the readability of the extracts. The co-authors' questions and comments on first translations have been valuable in doing this.

The organisation of the book

The opening chapter of the book introduces the premises of interaction research, which are located in the pioneering work of Erving Goffman, Harold Garfinkel and Harvey Sacks on human interaction and conversations. The chapter discusses the relevance of this work for social work interaction studies, offers basic tools for doing interactional analysis and describes briefly the various discursive research approaches on which interaction studies are anchored. It forms a methodological foundation for the following chapters concentrating on one key concept each.

The chapters of eight discursive and professional concepts – categorisa-tion, accountability, boundary work, narrative, advice-giving, resistance, delicacy and reported speech – are ordered according to their scope in relation to social work interaction. The starting concepts of categorisation and accountability are foundational for all social work interaction as for human interaction in general. Without creating categories and appealing to them or without accounting for certain behaviour or problems, social work would not even exist. Correspondingly the last two concepts, delicacy and reported speech, are more like features of social work interaction that might be (and in practice very often are) in use when, for example, doing categorisation or when accounting for certain behaviour.

All the key concept chapters follow the same structure. They (1) relate the concept to professional social work discussions, (2) present the origin of the concept in discourse studies, (3) review the social work relevant discourse literature where the concept has been applied and developed, (4) illustrate via data examples from naturally occurring interaction how the concept can be used when analysing social work interaction and (5) discuss its implications for social work practice. Each chapter, then, is both summative and empirical, introducing not only the concept, but an innovative approach to understanding that concept through the empirical analysis of face-to-face, naturally occurring talk. The concepts are often displayed simultaneously and connected to each other in real-life social work practices. So our data extracts could illustrate several of the concepts. We therefore make cross-references to the other chapters in order to demonstrate these connections.

In the final chapter, we summarise the main conclusions of the key concept chapters. Although we noted above that the primary aim of this volume is not to offer recipes of good communication, the implications for social work practice are still dealt with throughout the book. We strongly believe that interaction research can make an important contribution to social work practice, if not provide simple recipes. The final chapter discusses this topic as well as reflecting the forthcoming avenues and challenges of social work interaction research.

2

ANALYSING SOCIAL WORK INTERACTION

Premises and approaches

*Kirsi Juhila, Åsa Mäkitalo and
Martine Noordegraaf*

Where social workers meet clients, talk will be the main component of their relationship. Unlike most professions, social work is a profession of connecting conversations. In those conversations all kinds of different tasks are done and several goals are fulfilled. This is directly where institutional conversations depart from ordinary conversations. Institutional talk is not just regular talk but talk with a mission. From the social workers' point of view talk is the main vehicle for getting information from a client and for providing help and support where it is needed. All kinds of written reports and interprofessional meetings support that talk to complete a trajectory. From the clients' point of view talk is just as important; they describe their situations and problems and their needs for (or resistance to) support, account for and explain their behaviour and so on through verbal means. Without talk, social work could not be accomplished. This chapter introduces the premises for analysing social work conversations as institutional talk and attempts to demonstrate how studying talk-in-interaction increases our knowledge of what is at stake in this core practice of social work.

Conversations as the real-life laboratories of social work

Talk is not an individual act but always a joint endeavour. Professionals' and clients' social work talk in different situations (such as in multiprofessional case conferences, in meetings among social workers or in client–professional conversations) is directed at other participants and is also responded to by others. If understood as a joint endeavour, it follows that social work talk and the meanings it carries are seen to be created *in situ*. In other words, the participants' views, opinions and ideas are produced, developed and negotiated in conversations. Shotter (1993: 2) uses the concept of conversational realities when referring to this construction *in situ* and writes:

> instead of focusing immediately upon how individuals come to know the objects and entities in the world around them, we are becoming more interested in how people first develop and sustain certain *ways* of relating themselves to each other in their talk, and then, from within these ways of talking, make sense of their surroundings.

In social work conversations the participants make sense of clients' situations, problems, future prospects and the available supporting and helping methods and tools. In this regard these conversations have realities of their own; they are the *real-life laboratories of social work*.

In this book the focus is on these real-life laboratories. Accordingly, we analyse how social work interaction proceeds in different real-life settings and concentrate on the participants' ways of making sense of these settings 'without being shackled by normative standards of "good" communication' (Silverman 1997: 27) and without rushing to extra-situational explanations of the settings. As Silverman (1997: 23–25) reminds us, researchers should avoid treating people as 'puppets' (who just follow structural or psychological determinants) or 'dopes' (researchers know better).

In the following, we aim to orient readers to the bases of research that concentrates on conversational realities of social work and which approaches them as real-life laboratories. We start by introducing Erving Goffman's ideas of the interaction order and one of the cornerstones of Harold Garfinkel's ethnomethodology, namely members' methods. These influential micro-sociological developments form a basis for analysing social work conversations as domains of their own. After that we illustrate the interaction order and members' methods in action by using one piece of social work conversation as an example. In the discussion of this piece of conversation we pay special attention to:

1   Sequentiality, meaning the temporal organisation of interactants' talk or, in other words, how utterances such as questions, offers and hints always come in pairs with responses of all kinds. Talking together involves responding to one another.
2   Other features of institutional interaction that are used in subsequent chapters, which examine in detail special characteristics of conversational realities and their accomplishments in social work interaction (e.g. accountability, advice-giving, resistance, etc.).

The chapter ends with a short description of the research approaches that are useful in social work interaction studies.

The interaction order and members' methods

In this book we draw on the research tradition established by Goffman, especially his theory of the interaction order. Goffman (1983: 2) promoted the face-to-face domain as analytically viable, 'a substantive domain of its own right'. By this he meant that this domain should be studied using micro-analytical methods that take into consideration and make visible the rules of interactional organisation itself. From this it follows that the events in an interactional domain cannot be interpreted by explaining them in terms of outside factors (such as economic structure) or internal factors (such as psychological reasons). In the interaction order it is not enough to describe people as social workers or clients; they become social workers or clients through their talk and interaction. In this approach, macro issues or personal (psychological) issues are not neglected but are studied as embedded in interaction. Heritage (2001: 48) writes:

> Social interaction, he [Goffman] argued, embodies a distinct moral and institutional order that can be treated like other institutions, such as the family, education, religion etc. . . . it comprises a complex set of interactional rights and obligations, which are linked both to 'face' (a person's immediate claims about 'who s/he is' in an interaction), more enduring features of personal identity, and also to large-scale macro social institutions.

The interaction order is both deeply *moral* and *relational*. This is to say that, once individuals encounter each other, the norms of interaction are always present and in use. Individuals expect each other to behave in anticipated and jointly acceptable ways, which creates the basis for moral order. The moral order of interaction is not context bound, but similar norms, such as the expectation that individuals take turns of talk in a certain order, are present wherever people interact with each other. Violations of the norms are possible, but when individuals recognise violations as exceptions from the norms they simultaneously reproduce the norms and the moral order of interaction. For instance, if you do not receive an answer from a person to whom you have asked a question (a violation of the norm/an exception to the norm), you might repeat the question. If you still do not get a response, you are entitled to start accounting for the missing answer – for example, you might wonder whether the question was not heard or was too difficult for the other person to respond to (acts of recognising the violation). These interactional rules are the basis of communication and can be seen in use from a young age. It is remarkable how young children learn not only to speak grammatically correctly but how they also 'grasp' the interactional order. People with communication problems however, such as autism, have great difficulties with relationships, partly due to the fact that they do not grasp the interaction order.

As in the citation by Heritage above, interactional rights and obligations implement the moral order. In face-to-face conversations individuals' (relational) rights and obligations are often bound together. Individuals have a right and an obligation to talk and to be heard when their personal matters are discussed; they have a right and an obligation to make proposals when somebody has presented a problem needing a solution; and so on. Explaining and accounting for the violations of interactional norms can also be seen as rights and obligations. This relates to Goffman's (1955) ideas of *face* and *face work*. If the individual does not offer any solution to a personal problem presented by someone, s/he might instead provide an explanation for not doing that ('I really don't know, I am struggling with the same problem myself'). By doing so, s/he can save her/his face by presenting herself/himself as a caring person in spite of not offering any solution. The individuals can also save each other's faces in the interaction by reasoning why they do not fulfil their interactional obligations ('she is not able to help you now, because of her own situation'). In addition to interactional rights and obligations, face work displaying the moral order of interaction often links to delicate topics. If the topics threaten to embarrass or to stigmatise someone present, the individual concerned (or others) might, for instance, soften or ignore the topic or make excuses.

Furthermore, Heritage notices that the interaction order, as Goffman understood it, is linked to the *enduring features of personal identity* and to the more *macro-scale social institutions*. These are important issues to be considered in analysing social work interaction. When clients and social workers discuss, for instance, concerns related to clients' lives, there are often longer-term and more enduring identity issues present than just 'here and now' roles. One party might have a long history as a child protection client, for instance as 'a parent who is not coping', and the other party as a child protection worker, as 'an experienced professional'. Although not treated as unchangeable or fixed, these kinds of longer-term identity constructions display important roles in social work interaction order. 'The experienced professional' who has known 'the parent who is not coping' for a long time might start the discussion with an accusation about the latest failure of the parent and can demand explanations or give advice. Correspondingly, an interaction is created in which the parent is expected to explain the failure and to accept the advice, which would be inappropriate had other identities been in play.

Social work in itself is a macro-scale social institution with its own rules and norms; it is societal change, helping and controlling work with certain tasks and missions (e.g. to protect children). In such interaction, social work as a social institution is always strongly present in the acts of individuals, which cannot be ignored when analysing this interaction. However, the focus of analysis should still be on participants' orientation, on *members' methods*, when analysing interaction. Macro-scale social institutions or other 'social structures' only become relevant in the course of conversations if the participants involved make them relevant, that is, talk them into being. Researchers should 'discover them in the members' worlds, if they are there' (Schegloff 1992: 128).

Like Goffman, Garfinkel was interested in how individuals create social and moral order when interacting with each other in various settings (see Heritage 1984). He named individuals as cultural members, which emphasises their shared actions and active roles in this creation. He (Garfinkel 1967: 1) wrote: 'that the activities whereby members produce and manage settings of organized everyday affairs are identical with members' procedures for making those settings "account-able"'.

According to Garfinkel, members' methods in making settings 'account-able' should be the focus of research. It is not satisfactory to explain those situations by claiming that members just invoke some general rules (Garfinkel 1967: 32–33). Focusing on members' methods is the core idea of ethnomethodology, originated by Garfinkel. The concept of ethnomethodology includes the words *ethno* and *method*, referring to the methods produced and used by ordinary people (members) in everyday life. Jayyusi (1991: 234) succinctly defines what it means to concentrate on members' methods in ethnomethodological research:

> Rather than giving accounts and explanations of members' conduct, values, beliefs and judgements, it [ethnomethodology] analytically examines the ways that conduct, belief and judgement are organised, produced and made intelligible in members' own accounts and descriptions, and how they are embedded in various other practices. The accounts are treated as features of those practices, the descriptions as constituents of conduct.

Following this definition the gaze of research is directed to the situated activities themselves. Members' methods are part of those activities, not separate from them (Francis and Hester 2004: 28). In practical terms members' methods can be approached by analysing how participants orient to each other's actions and to the settings in question. When studying face-to-face social work conversations, this requires that one should make visible how the participants make the settings account-able: how they describe the settings in question, what topics they select to be discussed, what kinds of tasks, decisions and roles they orient to and so on. So, an analyst in this tradition needs good eyes and ears to observe what is going on in the interaction, trying not to predefine or to interpret what is going on or what is in people's minds. The focus of analysis is on how people talk and about what. Having said that, there is of course a world beyond interaction related to settings, history and mentality. We can add knowledge from the context of the interaction by interviewing the members of conversation or by reading texts on the background of both people and situations, but these only function as help in analysing the interaction.

The interaction order in action

We now present a short example of the real-life laboratory of social work. The aim is to highlight the presence of the interaction order and members' methods in everyday social work face-to-face conversations and to show the implications of this approach for research. The conversation is located in a low-threshold outpatient substance abuse clinic targeted at clients who suffer from serious drug abuse problems. The clinic is situated in a large Finnish town. The client is in his thirties. He is about to start a new phase in his life because, after many years of homelessness and living in several institutions, he has a rental flat of his own, accompanied by regular support in his home (known as floating support). The extract of conversation is part of a case conference whose participants are the client (C), a social worker from the clinic (P1) and a professional (P2) working in the floating support. Although this is a special case and conversation, it also carries many general features of social work conversations, as we can see (see the transcription symbols in the Appendix on page 181):

```
 1   P1:   is there something that should be taken into account now so that your
 2         housing would then be successful? it is indeed an excellent thing that you
 3         will get your very own rented flat in xxx ((name of a neighbourhood))
 4         it is really fantastic when thinking that you have been living for four
 5         five years in different institutional housing places (2) in rather heavy
 6         [places.
 7   P2:   [mmm
 8   P1:   Anno ((name of the place)) and and that Venno's ((name of the place))
 9         psychiatric ward for substance abusers and (3) the shelter for homeless
10         people and (3) Latoma ((name of the place)) and (4)
11   P2:   yeah it would be good to know right at the beginning at this preparation
12         phase what are those concerning or what concerns we should
13         seriously seek to solve together and to think how to get over them and
14         different tools and alternatives (2)
15   C:    well nothing comes to my mind other than (1) if I possibly
16         [relapse and so
17   P2:   [yeah what happens to you then? how does it start? how fast
18         does it progress and what is it like when it starts?
19   C:    (7) well I am then pretty mixed-up all the time you can't avoid noticing
20         it
21   P2:   would you answer phone calls (.) when thinking for instance that our
22         activities run so that we of course make agreements on how one
```

```
23        ((refers to clients)) participates in groups and in which groups and
24        in the beginning of course the participation is pretty intensive and in
25        addition there are weekly home visits and when these relapses occur
26        then we might have difficulties to contact some clients then we
27        have great difficulties in acting (1) it sort of delays that we might not
28        manage to intervene that is what I meant when asking whether we
29        are able to contact you
30        would you answer ((your phone)) and tell us what's going on?
31   C:   (6) well I really have to think about [that
32   P1:                                        [ymm
33   P2:                                           [yeah it is really important that
34        (1) it is
35   C:   I think I will answer [but it depends a bit on my mood ((at the moment)).
36   P2:                        [yeah
37   P2:  yes I think that these would be extremely important agreements to be
38        able to make that whatever the mood and condition is we could contact
39        you and start thinking what could we begin to do now (1) it is a rather
40        exciting situation to start living on you own after such a long time
41   P1:  mmm
42   P2:  so feeling nervous that is rather wise really to anticipate what if a
43        relapse comes what happens then (1) but it has to be considered how to
44        act in different situations (1)
45   C:   yes
46   P2:  so the way we act ((starts describing the institutional practices of
47        the floating support generally in cases of relapses))
```

If we just look at the first turns of the conversation (lines 1–16), it tells us rather easily what business is going on here. The first speaker raises the topic: what issues should be taken into account when one of the participants in the conversation moves to a flat of his own to ensure that this new housing state will be successful. The other speaker develops the topic by defining the issues as possible concerns related to this new situation. Both of the first speakers address their words to the third participant ('your housing', 'you will', 'what concerns you'), who also responds to the first turns by starting to consider the possible concerns (lines 15–16). The first turns of talk clearly show that this conversation is a joint endeavour. The participants orient to each other's talk and to the topic selected by the first speaker. This orientation displays the interaction order and its moral character, since the participants draw on certain shared interactional norms. The first speakers direct their words to the third participant by formulating questions about his personal future. Following the moral order of interaction, the respondent answers the questions. He has both the right and the obligation to do so, especially when the questions deal with his personal matters and future. Not answering at all without an appropriate explanation would easily be interpreted as a violation of the interaction order and would threaten the face of the questioners. However, there is another dimension of face (saving) present at the beginning of the conversation. This relates to a suspicion alluded to in the conversation that the respondent will perhaps not manage his housing successfully in the future and thus might become stigmatised as an incompetent person. The first speakers display this face-threatening orientation of their talk, where they emphasise that a big change (moving to your own flat after several years of homelessness and living in institutions) can understandably produce some coping difficulties. They also show readiness to share the possible concerns in this big life change (the 'we talk' on lines 12–14).

The enduring features of personal identities and macro-scale social institutions, which are linked to the interaction order (Heritage 2001: 48), are present at the beginning of the conversation. When relating themselves to each other the participants simultaneously make sense of their history and surroundings (Shotter 1993: 2). The first speaker indicates the enduring personal features when she refers to the respondent's five-year history of homelessness, including periods in a psychiatric hospital. The respondent is implicitly categorised as a person with housing and mental health problems. 'Knowing' these enduring problems is connected to the speaker's own history (and to her enduring features of personal identity). In her first turn she implies that she has known the respondent for some time already and has perhaps even witnessed his path through five years of homelessness. This 'knowing' makes her entitled to talk and ask about the respondent's future and concerns related to housing (cf. moral order).

So far we have called the participants of this conversation speakers, questioners and a respondent. However, some macro-scale institution is clearly present in the interaction. We easily interpret the turns as presented by kinds of professionals (questioners) and a service user or a client (the respondent). The features of social work interaction are clear: discussion revolves around possible concerns and problems; different tools for helping and problem solving alternatives are promised to be available if the concerns are realised. The questioners seek serious cooperation with the respondent in this promising but also vulnerable situation of change.

Above we have demonstrated how the participants themselves orient to the enduring personal features and macro-scale social institutions and talk them into being in the conversation. This is what concentrating on the interaction order and on the members' methods means. Researchers should not seek extra-situational explanations for the conversations, nor try to get inside people's heads to find reasons for their talk. In the following we look more closely at two important aspects of the interaction order relevant to studying social work conversations, namely sequentiality and the features of institutional interaction. We illustrate these aspects using the example of conversation displayed above.

Sequentiality

Ethnomethodological studies of talk-in-interaction have been developed by creating concepts and tools to analyse the orderliness of social actions in naturally occurring real-life conversations. The pioneer of this developing work is Harvey Sacks, whose findings created the basis for the research tradition called *conversation analysis*, also known as micro-sociology (Sacks 1972b, 1992; Sacks *et al.* 1974). The notion of *sequentiality*, meaning temporal ordering of turns of talk, is one of Sacks's key findings. He 'noticed that what speakers do in their next turns is related to what prior speakers do in the immediate prior turns' (Psathas 1995: 13). This often relates to a 'current speaker selects next' technique, wherein the speaker designs his/her words for a certain recipient who then has a right and an obligation to respond (Sacks *et al.* 1974: 704). Furthermore, as Heritage and Atkinson (1984: 9) note, 'just as a second speaker's analysis and treatment of the prior is available to the first speaker, so it is also available to overhearers of the talk, including social scientists'. It is the members' methods that are in use and the focus of interest here. The recipients of the prior turns analyse information embedded in the turns and display some interpretative conclusions of their own in the following turns of talk (Heritage and Atkinson 1984: 8). This is exactly what is happening in our example. The floating service professional displays in her turn (lines 11–14) an orientation to the immediate prior turn presented by the clinic social worker: she agrees with the social worker that the change situation demands discussion about the issues that should be taken into account in the future (the turn starts with the word 'yeah') and reformulates these issues as concerns. The professionals clearly also 'select' the client as the next speaker. Accordingly, the client recognises this 'selection', since he takes a turn and relates it to the immediate prior turns of the professionals. He displays his conclusion of these turns visibly, by raising one possible concern (lines 15–16). Similar sequentiality – the speakers' orientation to the prior turns and the reformulations or interpretative conclusions of the turns in the next turns – can be read throughout the example.

One of the basic structures of temporal sequentiality is called *adjacency pairs*. Adjacency pairs are at least two turns long and have at least two parts (Psathas 1995: 18). One pair always goes before the other, as in greeting–greeting, question–answer, suggestion–acceptance/rejection, request–acceptance/rejection, complaint–excuse/justification pairs (Silverman 2007: 66). Adjacency pairs are both temporarily related (one goes before the other) and 'discriminatively' related (since the first pair implicates what is the appropriate next pair) (Psathas 1995: 18; Silverman 2007: 66–67). This relates closely to the interaction order as the moral order (to speakers' rights and obligations). Participants in interaction expect questions to be answered or greetings to be responded to. The absences, or even short delays, of the second pairs or 'wrong' second parts are noticed and can be treated as indicators of some sort of interactional trouble (Psathas 1995: 18). Our example includes three question–answer adjacency pairs. The first one starts on lines 1–14, where the professionals make a sort of joint question to the client about issues/concerns to be taken into account when he moves to his own flat. The client gives an answer, an appropriate second part on lines 15–16. The second question–answer pair is on lines 17–20: the professional asks what the relapse is like, and the client answers by describing it (lines 19–20). The long pause before the answer indicates that the second part is expected by the prior speakers. The third pair begins on line 21 with the professional's question of whether the client would answer the phone during his possible forthcoming relapses. The client's answer is to be read from line 31 onwards. In addition to these three question–answer pairs, the last part of the conversation has elements of a suggestion–acceptance pair. There the professional underlines the importance of making an agreement on how they (the professionals in the floating support service) can contact the client, even during possible relapses (lines 37–44). By responding with 'yes' (line 45), the client displays acceptance of this suggestion.

There are no obvious signs of interactional troubles or inappropriate or absent second pairs in this conversation. However, the uncertain answer to the first question might indicate some slight trouble. The client does not answer directly to the question but displays some hesitation ('well nothing comes to my mind other than . . .', line 15) which might not be seen as an appropriate answer. However, the professional's immediate positive minimal response (line 17) strengthens the appropriateness of the client's answer. Other signs of possible interactional troubles are the client's delayed answers (lines 19 and 31). However, these can be interpreted to be more like thinking pauses; the client himself begins one delayed answer, after a long pause, by saying 'well I really have to think about' (line 31).

Preference organisation is another important element of sequentiality and also implicates the moral order of conversations. Preference organisation means that the first turn sets up 'normative expectations on what is to follow' (Antaki 2011: 2). This is linked to adjacency pairs, for instance it is preferable to accept an invitation or a suggestion than to reject it. In the latter case (rejection) the second parts usually include some sort of account for the unexpected response. Preference organisation might also be constructed so that first turns imply 'preferred' kinds of second turns, such that the question 'So you are quite happy now?' implies a 'yes' answer (Silverman 1998: 123). In our social work conversation this kind of implication is present in the professional's last turn (lines 37–44), which produces an expectation that the client will agree with the content of the suggestion (the need to make an agreement). With his 'yes' answer the client follows this normative expectation.

Sequentiality is not reduced to relations between turns that immediately precede and follow each other. It is also clear that 'long and complex sequences can be built *around* a single adjacency pair through what Schegloff (2007) calls *expansions*' (Peräkylä *et al.* 2008b: 15). These expansions or extended sequences might be in service of *telling stories* in conversations (Psathas 1995: 21). In social work conversations joint storytelling is often the case when discussing, for example, clients' problems, their history, their present stage and their future prospects. Our example contains some elements of storytelling when the social worker starts her opening turn by describing the client's past and then turns her gaze to his future, living in his own flat. Furthermore, Silverman (1998: 108–109) notices that according to Sacks's *'chaining rule'* participants can produce, for instance, several question–answer pairs that constitute a long chain in one conversation. The chain develops when the original questioner uses his/her right to speak by asking for clarification or more information, seeking questions after having received the answers to the prior questions. This kind of Q–A–Q–A chain, sequences of sequences, can be called the *interview format*, which is usual in a certain kind of professional–client settings (Silverman 1997: 41–45; 1998: 108–109). In our social work conversation the participants accomplish exactly this kind of a chain. The professionals ask altogether three questions, the last two of which are clarifying or information-seeking questions based on the client's prior answers (What is the relapse like? Would the client answer the phone during relapses?). Another typical chain in social work conversation is the alternation of the professional's information-delivering turns (often including giving advice) and the client's information-receiving turns, which Silverman (1997: 41–45) calls the *information delivery format*. When looking at our example this format begins in the professional's last three turns, where she stops questioning and moves on to delivering information on why having a common plan – if relapses occur – is so important in this new and exciting situation and then continues to describe the general practices of the floating support (lines 33–34, 37–44 and 46–47).

In addition to the expansions in the same conversation, sequences can be produced so that they are connected with past encounters (Peräkylä *et al.* 2008b: 15). The participants in the present conversation might have a history of joint conversations. They have perhaps talked about similar topics or problems before. However, when the focus is on the members' methods, this history of encounters is relevant only if it is talked into being by one or several participants in the present conversation. In our example the social worker makes the history relevant and noticed (lines 1–10). The conversation does not begin from zero; the professional constructs the client's history 'as a client' as an important starting point for this encounter. Although she does not refer directly to the previous conversations with the client, it indicates that the client's history is something that has been discussed before.

Features of institutional interaction

Although Goffman saw the interaction order as a domain in its own right, he did not deny its links to large-scale social institutions (Heritage 2001: 48). As discussed earlier in this chapter, social work in itself can be regarded as a large-scale social institution, which is culturally known for its helping, supporting, controlling and change work tasks. Social work is done in several settings, which have specific societal and institutional duties and missions, in addition to the general social work tasks. Relying on the members' methods approach we do not assume that the participants in social work conversations follow these social work tasks and specific institutional duties and missions automatically, like puppets. Instead, we are interested in the ways they are present in social work interaction: do the participants make them real and, if so, how? Or do they perhaps resist them and, if so, how? When doing this kind of an analysis, Heritage's (1997: 106; see also Drew and Heritage 1992a: 21–25) list of the features of institutional interaction is useful:

1 The interaction normally involves the participants in specific goal orientations that are tied to their institutional-relevant identities: doctor and patient, teacher and student, bride and groom, and so on.
2 The interaction involves special constraints on what will be treated as allowable contributions to the business at hand.
3 The interaction is associated with inferential frameworks and procedures that are particular to specific institutional contexts.

The first feature links the specific *goals* of the institutional settings and relevant *identities* together. It is easy to add the social worker–client pair to the list of institutional identity pairs. In our example the participants orientate notably to this pair and its reciprocal identities. The goal orientation tied to the identities is also present in the interaction. The overall goal in the conversation is to ensure that the client's move to live independently is successful. The social worker evokes this goal in the first turn (lines 1–2). At the same time, with this goal setting, she produces the institutionally relevant social worker identity for herself; she is the one whose duties involve supporting the client to reach the goal. The other professional shares this worker identity when she presents herself as a person who is in a position to offer 'different tools and alternatives' that help in achieving the goal (lines 11–14). It is interesting how the professional uses 'we' in her talk. She counts both the workers and the client to be the same 'we group' who share the same goal and thus collaborate to reach it (lines 12–14). In spite of this 'we talk' the workers create different obligations. The relevant client identity includes disclosing possible concerns that might endanger the successful housing (lines 1–2 and 11–12). The client identity includes also being the one who receives help and support (and control) from the workers. In this sense, the identities of the workers and the client are reciprocal (Juhila and Abrams 2011). Reciprocal identities such as these are not equal but more or less *asymmetrical*, which is common in such institutional identity pairs in which the professional expertise of one party is present and used over the other party.

The client orients to the identity that the professionals (as experts) create for him. This can be read from his answers, in which he discloses relapsing as a possible concern (lines 15–16), explicates it (lines 19–20) and participates in creating the plan in case he relapses (lines 31 and 35). The professionals for their part support this appropriate 'client talk' with minimal responses (lines 17, 33 and 36) and feedback (lines 33–34). However, the client shows uncertainty as to whether he is able to follow the plan (answering the workers' phone calls) during a possible relapse (lines 31 and 35). This kind of uncertainty can be regarded as belonging to the client identity in the transition situation, where the client is defined as still on his way to reaching the goal (successful housing and leaving the identity of a client). The floating support professional shows acceptance of this uncertainty but at the same time accomplishes her institutional identity obligations by encouraging and motivating the client to follow the plan (to agree with it), heading towards more independent living (lines 37–44).

The second feature of institutional interaction – namely *special constraints* – relates to the first, since the goals and relevant identities also reflect the constraints on what will be treated as allowable contributions in certain settings and the business at hand. Constraints can be oriented as powerful and legally enforceable, and as local and negotiable (Drew and Heritage 1992a: 23–24). These two ways of orientation have a dynamic relationship, and their simultaneous presence is productive for institutional intervention. However, the orientations have different emphases depending on the institutional context. The more local and negotiable orientation is in use in our social work conversation. The professionals talk into being the institutional task of supporting and controlling the client on his way towards more independent housing and living. There are two institutional settings present in the conversation, namely the low-threshold substance abuse clinic (P1) and the floating support (P2), which both work with adult clients whose clienthood is voluntary. The workers orient to this 'voluntary nature' of the encounter by asking questions and making suggestions to the client and by persuading him to cooperate with them without making any references to coercive actions or tools (which could be regarded as non-allowable in this setting). The client orientates to the situation accordingly. More powerful and enforceable social worker orientation can be accomplished, for instance in hospital admissions where the social workers might justify sometimes very strong interventions in the lives of clients by referring to their legal obligations (in this setting interfering could be regarded as allowable).

The third feature related to *inferential frameworks and procedures* is not independent from the above two features either. In accomplishing the institutionally relevant identities the participants simultaneously position themselves towards inferential frameworks and procedures that are particular to the institutional contexts in question. Constraints are also embedded in these frameworks and procedures. Social work interaction associates often with professional inferential frameworks, such as understanding social work as a well-planned, client-centred process of change or as interventions in trouble situations and behaviour. Specific institutional contexts also invite more or less strict procedures regarding interaction, for example expectations to create activation plans in job centres based on ready-made forms with questions and tick boxes. This third feature can also be formulated as the presuppositions of institutional interaction. For instance, it is presupposed that the institutional representative can operate as a 'change officer', asking whether and how change appears in a client's life. It also legitimates the asymmetry in the relationship, where a change officer enquires about personal and private aspects of a client's life. Such an entrance is normally not resisted in institutional communication because it is part of the institutional logic that 'explains' behaviour that would be considered odd in an ordinary, non-institutional situation. Another presupposition is about knowledge: it is assumed that the change officer knows about change and that the client lacks such knowledge. Presuppositions are heavily relied upon and attended to in institutional conversations. They are often consequential for how the participants go about their interaction in terms of what are considered relevant topics that need to be attended to and how 'activities' within the conversation are sequentially organised to meet the expected outcome (what is to be achieved in an institutional sense).

The general inferential framework on which the participants in our example seem to draw, directed by the workers, seems to be this change orientation, which is a common framework in social work and also is supported by the goals of institutional communication. This change orientation is displayed in the first turn (lines 1–6), where the client is defined as being in transition from homelessness towards more independent living in his own flat. The following interview format used in the conversation also associates with particular, change-oriented procedures in this special institutional setting. Question–answer sequences concentrate on the issues that might support or prevent the ultimate goal of successful change. The professionals' information delivery about this kind of a transition situation in general (what is to be expected and what kinds of difficulties should be prepared for) is in line with the change orientation too.

Approaches to interaction analysis

In this chapter we have introduced the premises of research that approaches conversations as real-life laboratories of social work. We have illustrated what it means to analyse social work conversations as morally ordered interaction and from the point of view of members' methods. Special attention has been paid to the sequentiality and the institutional features of interaction. The roots of the research tradition focusing on conversational realities are found first of all in Goffman's writings, in Garfinkel's ethnomethodology and in Sacks's notions on the orderliness of naturally occurring conversations. In addition to the work of these pioneers there are other early influences as well, such as Wittgenstein's (1953) ideas on language games, Bakhtin's (1981) analyses of dialogical voices and Austin's (1962) speech act theory.

First of all we have presented such aspects of Goffman's, Garfinkel's and Sacks's work that are useful in studying social work interaction and are in use in this book. Hence, this chapter is not to be read as an overall introduction to Goffman's, Garfinkel's and Sacks's work. We are also well aware that these pioneers' and their successors' researches differ somewhat from each other. For instance, Goffmanian analysis and conversation analysis relying on Sacks's innovative findings have quite different agendas. The former underlines the moral implications of interactional patterns and their social consequences, while the latter puts more emphasis on how conversations unfold and on participant orientation in 'here and now' interaction. While recognising these differences we have, however, attempted to show how productive and relevant elements can be retrieved from these different ways of approaching interaction when analysing social work conversations.

The early pioneers' research on interaction and on members' methods have influenced several closely related approaches during recent decades. This expansion of interaction analysis is part of the phenomenon that is called discursive or linguistic turn in social sciences. The turn has meant that the practices and realities of talk, texts and interaction have been the subject for research in different ordinary life and institutional settings. These approaches include conversation analysis (CA), membership categorisation analysis (MCA), discursive psychology (DP), critical discourse analysis (CDA) and narrative analysis (NA). CA and MCA are both based on Sacks's (1992) empirical and methodological work. The origin of DP lies in the writings and studies by Potter, Wetherell and Edwards (e.g. Potter and Wetherell 1987; Edwards and Potter 1992; Potter 1996; Edwards 1997), whereas CDA often dates back to Foucault's texts (e.g. 1981, 1986). In comparison to the others, NA is a more scattered research approach but, from the point of view of social work, the writings of Hall (1997) and Riessman (2008), as well as of Gubrium and Holstein (2009), are important.

The 'second-generation' approaches listed above are used with different emphases in the following chapters focusing on the specific aspects of social work interaction. None of the chapters relies purely on one approach. Instead, the elements of approaches are applied when they are regarded as relevant from the point of view of the interactional concept under study.

The most applicable elements of the different approaches in relation to social work studies can be shortly listed as being the following. As was already indicated in this chapter, CA offers tools to analyse social work conversations on a turn-by-turn basis (sequentiality). The importance of MCA lies in its methods of making visible the power of cultural categories and categorisations in human relations – how they are talked into being and used in consequential ways in different encounters (Jayyusi 1984; Hester and Eglin 1997). In social work interaction categorisation often relates to clients' identity categories and an interest in what actions are done with these identity categories (see Stokoe 2009). DP addresses how psychological matters are constructed, displayed and responded to when people interact in everyday and institutional situations (Potter 2012). This approach is useful, since psychological matters are no doubt present in many occasions in social work conversations, for example in talk about inner states of mind or in accounting for certain behaviour or troubles. CDA brings in the analysis of power relations and the entanglement of power and knowledge to social work interaction studies (Fairclough 1992; Hall 2001). It also stresses the presence of larger-scale cultural discourses in 'here and now' encounters, including social work conversations. Lastly, different narrative analyses might benefit social work interaction studies in many ways. Social work conversations are often rich in stories, for example those related to the life stories of clients, to the causes of certain troubles or to the accounts of minor episodes.

3

CATEGORISATION

Åsa Mäkitalo

Plenty of textbooks dealing with social work concentrate on certain problems, such as mental health, violence, substance abuse or unemployment. To classify problems in such terms is foundational for social work as a knowledge domain and is necessary for the ability to understand, discuss and intervene in identified problems. In this chapter, however, such classifications of problems are not taken as ready-made to be found and dealt with. Instead tools are provided to analyse how they are intrinsic to social work interaction as an institutional communicative practice and how both social workers and their clients are actively involved in their making. This requires an alternative approach and a set of questions that are more explorative in character: How do social workers and their clients come to talk about their concerns in terms of, for instance, 'neglect', 'learning disability' or 'physical abuse'? How do they arrive at a conclusion of what *kind* of problem they are dealing with? What consequences do these categories have in terms of intervention and action? What entitlements and obligations are implied for the parties involved? These are some of the issues to be raised when exploring categorisation in social work interaction.

Membership categorisation analysis

One scholar who early on took a profound interest in how categories work in interaction was the sociologist Harvey Sacks. The analytical work he pursued from the mid 1960s, as the reel-to-reel tape recorder allowed detailed analyses of naturally occurring conversations, was to systematically uncover how people – as cultural members – make themselves, others and their surroundings comprehensible to each other. So, instead of theorising about external social structure or internal individual characteristics to explain social problems, the work he pursued was to discover the ways in which people themselves *categorise to make sense* of people, events and actions in their local context (Hester and Eglin 1997). Sacks noted that 'a great deal of the knowledge that Members of a society have about the society is stored in terms of these categories' (1992: 40–41). As Sacks explains:

> [when] you get some category as an answer to a 'which'-type question, you can feel that you know a great deal about the person, and can readily formulate topics of conversation based on the knowledge stored in terms of that category.
>
> (1992: 40–41)

Many categories are what Sacks called *membership categories* – categories that describe people in terms of culturally identifiable groups. This means that, if someone presents herself as a 'single mother', your cultural knowledge about that membership category becomes a resource to draw on when continuing the conversation.

Categories in interaction accordingly *allow us to take things for granted*. When in use, some things need not be mentioned but are instead inferred. Sacks noted that sometimes membership categories come in *pairs*, such as 'husband' and 'wife'. Their existence is interdependent, which means that, if one is mentioned, the other is simultaneously made relevant without mentioning. So, if someone reports that a neighbour rescued the wife from a 'serious beating', we do not assume it is the neighbour's wife that has been beaten; neither do we assume that anyone could have beaten the wife. By using the category 'wife' when telling the story, her 'husband' is immediately alluded to as relevant to what is being told (i.e. as the one who performed the assault). Sometimes *collections* of categories are also alluded to in similar ways such that addressing someone as 'a sister' makes her 'family' relevant in the ongoing discussion.

Categories are, however, not only resources for understanding. We also *categorise to achieve something* in talk. Often, for instance, we want to make something particular relevant about another person (Edwards 1998). For example, to say that a person is a 'good liar' (Hester 1998) or a 'Hells Angels type' (Jayyusi 1984) when talking about problems with social relationships is not only a descriptive act. These categories seem to be crafted to achieve different things in such discussions. While the former is primarily invoked as an individual designator and alludes to the person as the source of trouble, the latter is crafted to make the membership of a social group relevant to the problems discussed. Categories to describe people and make certain things relevant about them seem to be readily at hand in everyday interaction, and in social work such categorisations enable the parties to sort out, negotiate and handle the problems they are concerned with.

As Sacks also noted, some membership categories are *activity-bound* and as such they are tied to certain entitlements and obligations for those involved. If a person, for instance, says that he is currently 'on parental leave' the category sets up expectations for both the professional and the client in the situation at hand. Their respective entitlements and obligations with regard to this category may then implicitly or explicitly be drawn on as resources in their encounter. Activity-bound categorisations are often prevalent in social work interaction when clients and professionals argue about rights and responsibilities. Let us take an example. While 'parents' in the everyday sense are ascribed responsibility for their children, they are usually not accountable for attending to them while 'at work'. If, however, a parent who is 'on parental leave' leaves his child unattended, this would not meet the expectations and activity-bound requirements; rather, the parent's non-attendance could potentially be categorised as 'ignorance' or 'neglect'. A particular parent may accordingly be questioned if activity-bound expectations are not met.

As Edwards (1991, 1998) notes, there are always alternative ways of describing people, events and actions. Categories have 'fuzzy membership boundaries and even contrasting possibilities for description' (Edwards 1991: 523). This means they do not only function to organise our under-standing of the world 'but are adaptable to the situated requirements of description' (p. 523). In commercials one might, for instance, hear 'I'm not only a dentist, I'm also a mother' – a description that is crafted to sell a particular product. In institutional practices such as social work, it is clear that categories are not only for talking (Edwards 1991). To categorise is an element of professional knowing and action as the social worker, for instance, investigates whether a child is 'at risk' (Hall *et al.* 2006; Hall and Slembrouck 2007). Many of the challenges and social dilemmas that social work is targeted to handle (i.e. poverty, delinquency, mental illness, neglect, abuse, addiction and prostitution to mention but a few) become salient when problems are to be defined, categorised and treated as a case of this or that 'kind'. Knowing just *how* to position oneself and categorise a case in insti-tutionally relevant ways is important to become recognised as a legitimate knower in interaction with clients and other professionals (Hitzler 2011). In institutional practices, categorisation initiates action and allows insti-tutional actors to intervene in people's lives. When analysing institutional categorisation a core analytic issue accordingly becomes the accountability at work in various activities and the outcomes and character for those involved (White *et al.* 2009).

Studies of categorisation in social work

In research, analyses of categorisation have contributed by highlighting many intriguing and important elements of social work practices. Such studies have provided insights into the process through which a person is transformed into a client of a particular kind. Such a process involves contributions at least from both the social worker and the persons involved and always implies some kind of transformation that may be more or less consequential for their everyday lives.

Several studies have taken an interest in how social workers and clients engage in joint activities to establish 'the case' through interaction. In vocational rehabilitation and guidance, for instance, the client is often expected to take an active role and contribute in the process of producing an individual action plan (Solberg 2011; Caswell *et al.* 2013). Other studies have analysed how institutional services become available, and how entitlements and obligations in providing and receiving services are negotiated among professionals and their clients in public employment offices (Mäkitalo 2003), in social welfare agencies (Linell and Fredin 1995; Hydén 1996) and in elderly care (Olaison and Cedersund 2006; Olaison 2010).

Other studies have focused on the construction of clienthood (Hall *et al.* 2003). To become a 'good' client, for instance, seems to require that the person take on the institutional perspective of his or her own situation. This seems to be the case whether it concerns children with difficulties in school or adults with difficulties in finding a job (Hjörne and Mäkitalo 2008). There are also studies of how 'bad' clients are created and how transgressions of explicit or implicit norms of conduct might challenge the institutional agenda (Juhila 2003; Mäkitalo 2006). Clients sometimes resist the dominant categorisations of institutional actors such as the shelter residents in Juhila's study (Juhila 2004). Also, identities are negotiated through the construction of clienthood. Several studies have analysed what being a 'caring parent' or a 'responsible relative' implies, how expectations of such identities are gendered and when an intervention from the institution is considered necessary (Paoletti 2001; van Nijnatten and Hofstede 2003; Virokannas 2011).

Studies have also been conducted that focus on how established institutional categories are assessed or matched against a particular case at hand (Baker 1997). Such studies are often illuminating when it comes to the daily workings of institutions that are often hidden from public view, for instance how persons are assessed for 'adoptive parenthood' (Noordegraaf 2008) or how 'students' become 'special students' (Mehan *et al.* 1986; Hjörne and Säljö 2012). The interactional work of categorising and classifying 'problems' is here a recurrent theme. Several studies of categorisation have also analysed how empirical observations along with professional judgements and tests, for instance, are adopted and used in the co-production of a 'factual' account that points to a particular diagnosis such as 'learning disabilities' or 'mental illness' (Smith 1978; Mehan 1993).

With such powerful means at their disposal, professionals are also incorporated into studies of categorisation with a focus on issues of accountability and the intricate interdependencies of institutions, professionals and their clients. What is required of them from other stakeholders has always been of great concern to professional organisations and specific requirements of efficiency and accountability need to be considered and balanced in relation to each case (Mäkitalo and Säljö 2002a; Hall and Slembrouck 2007; White *et al.* 2009; Saario and Raitakari 2010). In interagency work, for instance, professional membership and their activity-tied entitlements and obligations become boundaries that need to be both relied upon and negotiated as work is pursued (Hall *et al.* 2006).

When well established in a professional community categories are usually not challenged on a daily basis. Their peculiar force, sustainability and power lies in their use as adaptable means *to short cut* what have earlier been topics of deliberation, argumentation and reasoning. When established, such extensive discursive work is no longer necessary for people to be able to coordinate their actions and perspectives. When settled, categorisations are thus usually taken for granted, whether they are explicitly invoked or only alluded to in interaction. In the following I shall use a set of examples in order to make salient what an analysis of categorisation may illuminate when looking more closely at social work interaction. These examples are arranged so as to follow the process of social work, from how institutional membership is established to how a case is reported.

Exploring categorisation in interaction: data examples and analyses

Social work as a practice is enacted by interaction through text and talk. It does not happen just because there is an office, a social worker and a client visiting. Both parties usually need to enact their roles to some extent in order to establish their participation in the activity. I will begin with some examples of the ways institutional membership is initiated. The issue to consider is accordingly *how* relevant roles for social work are enacted implicitly or explicitly.

To establish institutional memberships

Our first set of examples is taken from an encounter at a social welfare office and an employment office in Sweden. The excerpts are taken from the very beginning of the encounters.

The 'social worker' and the 'client' as a category-pair

After a first greeting it usually takes just a few utterances to anticipate and initially establish the point of the meeting, to invite and accept institutional membership and to initiate the activity. This is exemplified with an extract from a social welfare agency where two persons (A and B) interact.

Extract 1 (from Hydén 2001)

1	A:	so you've come in order to apply for financial benefits
2	B:	yes
3	A:	since you came to see me
4	B:	yeah

The interaction in Extract 1 suggests that the participants assume a whole set of actions, arrangements, entitlements and obligations *in situ*. In turn 1, for instance, A formulates a conclusion as to what B wants, to be recognised and confirmed, rather than poses a question as to what kind of service B is seeking. The way A initiates the activity efficiently sets the agenda for their meeting and institutional memberships are simultaneously but tacitly suggested and accepted. How the conclusion was reached (as to what B wants) is explicitly noticed *as a recognisable action* 'since you came to see me'. By confirming this, B enters into an institutional relation with A, and their respective identities as institutional actors are enacted; B becomes an 'applicant' and A, the 'administrator' of his application. Both are interdependent; in Sacks's sense they constitute a *category-pair* and are *activity-bound*. In order for this to be comprehensible a set of inferences from the recognisable action needs to be made. First, it is noticeable that B came to see A (and not the opposite). Second, you do not randomly set up a meeting with A (when doing so you have some business in mind). Third, the particulars of the business are made evident by the fact that B came to see A (and not any employee at the welfare agency). Membership categories such as these may accordingly be implicitly enacted as in this case, since they rely on a whole set of institutional arrangements that these two interlocutors already know and are able to draw on. Sometimes, however, such membership category-pairs are also invoked explicitly, as in the following extract from a public employment office where a first encounter takes place between a vocational guidance officer and a job applicant.

Extract 2 (from Mäkitalo and Säljö 2002b)

1	Officer:	I'm Viola Vide[gren]
2	Applicant:	[yeah, I] got the
3		pa[pers]
4	Officer:	[and it-] I'm your, I'm [your]
5	Applicant:	[ye-]
6	Officer:	your new offi[cer]
7	Applicant:	[yes]
8	Officer:	here now, at the employment office
9	Applicant:	yes I got this other one from you
10	Officer:	yes

11	Applicant:	but nothing was written on [this]
12	Officer:	[no]
13	Applicant:	so I had to call here, and I nearly didn't get through
14		but then I got hold of a guy and then I got . . .
15	Officer:	yes, yes I'm so sorry [it's]
16	Applicant:	[no, but it's] no big deal
17	Officer:	((yawning:)) been a bit busy [I just]
18	Applicant:	[yes]
19	Officer:	put it in the envelope and sent it off
20	Applicant:	that easily happens
21	Officer:	without checking it properly
22	Applicant:	mm
23	Officer:	well, I asked you to visit me to meet you and hear
24		what your thoughts and plans [are]
25	Applicant:	[mm]
26	Officer:	and to see if there is something we can [help]
27	Applicant:	[mm]
28	Officer:	you with
29	Applicant:	now, I had fifty-two days left last Thursday
30		so now I must have forty-seven then
31	Officer:	mm
32	Applicant:	so that's a little more than two months [so]
33	Officer:	[mm]

What is interesting to note about this particular conversation between the vocational guidance officer, Viola, and the job applicant, Stig, is the way they quickly etablish their respective membership categories and get on with their business at a very early stage in their conversation. They do this without much elaboration or questioning, even though they have never met before. By invoking the institutional category 'officer' (line 6) in her greeting, Viola acknowledges her professional obligation to meet Stig in person 'to see if there is something we can help you with' (lines 26 and 28). Her use of the pronoun 'we' reveals that it is the employment office that takes an interest in Stig's 'thoughts and plans' (line 24). Stig does not, however, comment on his thoughts and plans. His response reveals that he is not a newcomer to this office. He immediately recognises the officer's account for a meeting as an invitation to discuss his current situation as a job applicant, and responds in terms of 'days left', which makes the issue of time limits salient to his current situation (line 29). Now, as 47 days amounts to 'a little more than two months' (line 32) we can conclude he is not referring to calendar days. Rather, Stig is describing his current situation as a job applicant in terms of the number of days left before his unemployment insurance expires. This restriction in time delimits not only the topic of their discussion, but also a set of available options to consider, which efficiently sets the agenda for their meeting.

Another thing that is implicitly at work in this conversation is the entitlements and obligations of the membership categories involved. As we can see in lines 2 and 3 Viola is interrupted by Stig even before he returns her initial greeting. Such interruption when meeting someone for the first time is unusual, but here it shows the importance and remarkable character of the event told – that some piece of information was missing on the written notice to attend. Viola acknowledges this problem and the extra efforts made by Stig, and provides an excuse (lines 15–19). What is at stake here, which only becomes salient when looking at the institutional arrangements, is their category-tied obligations and entitlements. By acknowledging the mistake (when omitting information on the form) Viola not only responds to the concern raised. She also acknowledges that she put the applicant in a situation where he was nearly not able to do what he is *institutionally obliged* to do – to show up when called for. As an officer, she is in this manner accountable for putting the applicant's entitlement to his unemployment insurance money at risk. In this case we see that their category-tied entitlements and obligations are interdependent and tacitly at work.

To make a case

As Goffman notes, '[s]ervers of all kinds have the right to ask those they serve for pertinent biographical information. To seek a service, then, is to expose oneself to questioning' (1983: 41). The information that is asked for by means of a textual form or in a face-to-face encounter needs to meet the particular arrangements of the institution in order to construct a case (i.e. something that the institution can work with). Clients' own stories, their concerns, their relations and their current situation are necessary descriptive elements when cases are made (see Chapter 6 on narrative). From what is reported, a process follows where *particular instances* of what is told and reported are taken into account as relevant for categorising the case – as a case of a certain kind. This means that the relation between the professional and the client is characterised by mutual interdependencies. This by no means suggests that their interaction is symmetrical. Asymmetry is usually a salient feature of any kind of professional–client interaction even if it is sometimes implicitly at work.

An instance of what? Moving from particular observations to categorisations

When it comes to social work interaction the client's situation and concerns are explored through the client's own story, but also other reports of earlier events (see Chapter 10 on reported speech) may be considered relevant for establishing and constructing a case. In the following we will see this kind of categorisation work in an encounter between a professional therapist and his client (a mother who is concerned about her son).

Extract 3 (from Bartesaghi 2009)

1	Therapist:	hmm. How do you know that there's something going on with him? How
2		can you tell?
3	Client:	I just think there's something going on, he's acting different.
4	Therapist:	what do you mean, different?
5	Client:	withdrawn from things.
6	Therapist:	has he always been withdrawn from things?
7	Client:	no.
8	Therapist:	it seems like a couple of years ago when you first came here in '93 he was sort
9		of sad and withdrawn. ((shows manila folder)) Here's his record.

The client is concerned that something is going on with her son. This kind of descriptive vagueness is typical of cases that have not yet been established. The therapist starts by asking *how the client knows* that something is going on (line 1), not taking the client's formulation at face value. At this stage the potential of a case is explored and the professional engages in questioning in order for them both to sort out what that 'something' means. Through the professional's questions (lines 1, 4 and 6) 'something' is characterised and specified in more concrete terms through descriptions of the son's action ('he's acting different', 'withdrawn from things'). Such observable features are accordingly reported as instances of something going on (a concern that potentially would call for a category of some 'kind' of trouble). The particular features of this description are recognised by the therapist and he shows that he keeps track of the family's earlier reported behaviour. By implicitly comparing the client's account to the case history, the claim that the son is acting differently as an indication of something is accordingly challenged and the concern may instead be redirected towards, for instance, the client's relation to her son.

Category contrasts in descriptions of deviance

While the former example showed how vaguely reported events are not pursued, but may instead be undermined by reference to earlier events reported, the next is an example of how category contrasts function in descriptions of people as being deviant from what is normatively expected. In this case a head teacher (HT) has a concern related to a child in school and brings it up with the educational psychologist (EP), who in turn recollects his memory of an earlier assessment of the same child that is made relevant to their conversation.

Extract 4 (from Hester 1998)

1	HT:	he's he's such a ahm you know so many children if they are telling you lies
2		you [it sta]nds out a [mile] the lying but with=
3	EP:	[mm] [mm]
4	HT:	=Robin
5	EP:	he's good
6	HT:	((sotto voce[1])) He's very good
7	EP:	he's quite I can't re[member the exact assessment]
8	HT:	[he's very good and so innoce]nt looking
9	EP:	yeah I seem to remember he's at least average intelligence isn't he?
10	HT:	oh yes about average [(1.5) something like that]
11	EP:	[he's not he's not ( ) no]
12	HT:	yeah yeah but er
13	EP:	yeah
14	HT:	he's a child you just can't tell whether he's lying or not
15	EP:	mm
16	HT:	most of the time I must admit I think he is lying but you try
17	EP:	mm
18	HT:	you would never get him to show it
19	EP:	mm

([1] Hester uses the musical term 'sotto voce', which means to intentionally lower the volume of one's voice for emphasis.)

In Extract 4 we can see how the professionals collaborate in comparing a particular boy with other children. This is done through contrasting 'so many children' (line 1) to the particular child 'but with Robin' (lines 2 and 4). Here the category is activity-bound (it concerns lying) and a distinction is implicitly established between what are recognisable as instances of normal lying among children in general (that 'stands out a mile', in line 2), while the opposite simultaneously becomes a relevant feature of Robin, implicitly separating his way of lying from the others. The category is further suggested through an individual designator that implies an extraordinary feature, 'he's good' (line 5), delivered by the educational psychologist, only alluding to the activity of lying that was introduced by the head teacher. The candidate category is then not only confirmed but clearly established by upgrading this feature of Robin as being 'very good' (line 6). As can also be noted, alternative categories are briefly considered by the educational psychologist as he recollects some earlier assessment of the child and mention of him being of 'average intelligence', but alternatives are directly dismissed and only alluded to ('he's not, he's not' in line 11). As Robin is identified as a 'very good liar' the point is not only to make such a description per se. Rather, the communication between child and adult is addressed in the interaction by the head teacher who 'just can't tell whether he is lying or not' (line 14) and a concern is raised of the risk to 'think he is lying' (line 16) most of the time.

Textual and narrative accounts in categorisation

Institutional membership categories, however, are not primarily descriptions of people themselves; they are more often co-products of specific institutional activities and priorities. They are productive in making 'cases' that are workable institutional tasks. In the encounter with established welfare arrangements, institutional categories and their potential interdependencies for coordinating actions and activities become salient. Such categories accordingly tend to penetrate local activities but also intervene in people's personal lives – to varying degrees and with different results. People's contact with an institution may, for instance, be based on free will, necessity or obligation, in which the range of flexibility in managing them will be displayed. For example, we enter, and leave, the category of 'train traveller' without much notice, while membership as a 'hospital inmate' or 'welfare recipient' requires to be worked up through extensive documentary procedures in order to achieve a distribution of entitlements, rights and obligations among the actors involved.

Institutional membership categories are accordingly consequential in both formal and informal ways and are also designed to move people to action. In the following example some extracts are used from an assessment of a child performed by a team of professionals and the mother of the child. While the mother's (MO) account of the child is based on her own observations in a home environment, the teacher's (SET) observations were drawn from classroom and school activities, and the psychologist's (PS) account was drawn from a set of tests used to assess the child. These different accounts are considered while making a case, and some of them play a more salient role than others.

Extract 5a: Part of the psychologist assessment of Shane (from Mehan 1993)

1	PS:	Shane is ah nine years old, and he's in fourth grade. Uh, he, uh, was referred
2		because of low academic performance and he has difficulty applying himself to his
3		daily class work. Um, Shane attended the Montessori School in kindergarten and
4		first grade, and then he entered Carlberg-bad in, um, September of 1976 and, uh
5		entered in our district in uh '78. He seems to have very good peer relationships but,
6		uh, the teachers, uh, continually say that he has difficulty with handwriting. 'kay.
7		he enjoys music and sports. I gave him a complete battery and, um I found that, uh,
8		he had a verbal IQ of 115, performance of 111, and a full scale of 115, so he's a

9		bright child. Uh, he had very high scores in, uh, information which is his long-term
10		memory. Ah vocabulary, was, ah, also, ah, considerably over average, good detail
11		awareness and his, um, picture arrangements scores, he had seventeen which is very
12		high=
13	SET:	=mmmm

After giving a brief description of the child's age and his grade in the school he attends at the moment, the psychologist quickly turns to the reason why a referral was made and why Shane is at all considered in need of assessing (lines 1–3). The reasons reported are poor academic performance and difficulties in applying himself to his daily class work, especially handwriting, with explicit reference to the teachers as having reported their concerns about this child (lines 6–7). The psychologist then moves on to refer to her own use of a battery of tests (lines 7–8), which have been given to Shane in order to assess his intellectual capacities. In the psychologist's rather extensive account (only the first part of which is displayed here) we can note a range of categories to measure such capacities and Shane is assessed accordingly. Framing her account in a psychologist's discourse, she identifies what a certain score on the scale indicates (lines 8–9). When reporting the results, the observations made are clearly mediated by the design of the tests and his performance is made salient *in relation to a norm* that places the child on a scale 'considerably over average' (line 10) on vocabulary, and 'very high' on information (line 9), which makes the psychologist conclude that 'he's a very bright child' with respect to these performance measures. Other measures were also reported, however, which gave him a standard score of 100, which compared with his overall score put him 'somewhat ah below his, you know, his capabilities' (Mehan 1993: 251). What is interesting to note here is that the results are reported as stable and appear as fixed when presented in numerical form.

Assessments such as these rely on statistical methods and procedures that make up (Hacking 1986) a 'generalised child', which emerge from the distribution of many observations of children. The deviations are placed at the margins of the normal distribution of observations (or in the 'tails' of what is referred to as the bell curve). Just where a score on the scale is regarded as a deviation from what's normal has accordingly already been decided upon and is a standardised measure. The kind of cultural knowledge that comes with this kind of well-established test battery is for many reasons very hard to challenge – it has been developed over more than a century by experts from several fields – and is here taken for granted and relied upon to say something about a particular child in a particular context. As the psychologist has reported her assessment she invites the others to provide information and the classroom teacher presents some conditions under which Shane has trouble, such as things that require fine motor skills, especially writing, and types of independent work, which are hard for him.

After a further discussion the psychologist asks the mother about her son's fine motor control at home. The special education teacher (SET) takes over this initiative and invites Shane's mother (MO) to contribute.

Extract 5b: Part of the mother's account of Shane (from Mehan 1993)

1	SET:	how do you find him at [home] in terms of using his fingers and fine motor
2		kinds of things? Does he do//
3	MO	=He will, as a small child he didn't at all. He was never interested in it, he
4		wasn't interested in sitting in my lap and having a book read to him, any things
5		like that//
6	SET	=mhmmm//
7	MO:	=which I think is part of it you know. His, his older brother was just the
8		opposite, and learned to write real early. Now Shane, at night, lots of times he
9		comes home and he'll write or draw. He's really doing a lot//
10	SET:	((inaudible))
11	MO:	=he sits down and is writing love notes to his girl friend (hehehe). He went in
12		our bedroom last night and turned on the TV and got out some colored pencils
13		and started writing. So he, really likes to, and of course he brings it all in to us
14		to see//
15	SET:	=mhmmm//
16	MO:	=and comment on, so I think, you know, he's not [NEGAtive] about//
17	SET:	=no//
18	MO:	=that anymore//
19	SET:	=uh huh
20	MO:	he was before, but I think his attitude's changed a lot

(// = denotes overlapping utterances)

As can be noted, the mother's account is markedly different from that of the psychologist, drawing on observations of Shane in a home enviroment where he chooses to engage in some things and not others (lines 3–5). The narrative describes a shift, over a longer period of time. By comparing earlier experiences of Shane 'as a small child' lacking interest (line 3) and contrasting that experience with 'Now' (line 8–9), when he is described as spontaneously and willingly engaging in writing and drawing (lines 11–13), a change in attitude is made relevant and emphasised (lines 13, 16 and 20). The account of the mother explicitly takes particular notice of positive signs of engagement when it comes to writing, displaying a trajectory that projects future developments. From this account only, we could come to the conclusion that the background of the reported concerns is not a sign or symptom of the category 'learning disability', but rather that the reported difficulties with writing are to be understood as transitory, against the backdrop of his history of not having been interested in writing until recently.

When categorisations of people are made in social work contexts, different kinds of accounts are drawn on. Some are experientially grounded in the richness of people's everyday lives and are presented through narratives and life histories (see Chapter 6 on narrative). The narrator can make relevant people's actions in many different ways: as intentional or accidental, as reactions to events or people, or as an unfortunate consequence of circumstance. In either case a narrative is told for the purpose of communicating what is considered relevant in the situation at hand from the perspective of the storyteller. In the mother's account, Shane is ascribed agency and as having an interest in writing and drawing (for the purpose of communicating with his girlfriend and getting some recognition from other family members). However, the psychologist's accounts based on classifications, standardised testing and descriptions of symptoms, which includes the observable 'trouble' with 'fine motor skills', were prevalent when categorising this case, even though there were competing versions and accounts provided from other professionals. As has been mentioned earlier, institutional membership categories are accordingly co-products of specific institutional activities and priorities. They are productive in making cases that are workable institutional tasks. This, accordingly, will have consequences for how a case is worked on, handled and pursued. Categories, when institutionally established, thereby call for action and intervention.

To intervene and move people to action

When a case is identified and categorised, there are certain entitlements and obligations for the parties involved that come into play in the interaction. Institutional texts, laws, rules and regulations may suddenly be made relevant in the interaction. Sometimes they are implicitly relied upon and only alluded to or hinted at (as in Extract 2); in other cases they are explicitly drawn on in the interaction. In the following examples we will see how activity-bound categorisations are drawn on to move the client to action.

Activity-bound entitlements and obligations

In the following example from Miller's (1991) study of a Work Incentive Program (WIN) office, this is a salient feature of the interaction. The staff member (SM) pursues the case by asking if the client engages in the category-relevant activity.

Extract 6 (from Miller 1991)

1	SM:	are you looking for work?
2	Client:	yeah, I have but I got a new car and it broke down. Besides, I don't have
3		enough money for gas. You can't drive without gas. I need the WIN money

4		for other things, living expenses
5	SM:	that's not what the money is for. It's for gas and other job search expenses
6	Client:	well, all I can say is, my kids come first. I'm gonna feed them before I go
7		lookin' for a job
8	SM:	what'll your kids do for food if you lose your grant? You will [lose the grant]
9		if you don't look for work

When asking 'Are you looking for work' (line 1), the staff member makes relevant the activity-tied nature of the institutional category 'job-seeker' in the interaction with the client. The category is already institutionally established so it does not have to be identified or even mentioned in this case. It is accordingly taken for granted, but it is enacted and made relevant to the situation at hand as the interlocutors meet. By asking, the case and the task is accordingly initiated, but the particular way the question is formulated as an open question rather than one that takes the category-tied activity for granted (such as 'How is your job search going?') suggests that it is crafted to be heard as a form of questioning. The client responds by confirming, but is visibly challenged as an account is provided of his current situation, which makes relevant some trouble in pursuing the activity as expected (lines 2–4). This account further displays the client's need for some additional support in order to be able to proceed with the activity. The staff member now draws on the category-tied obligations (i.e. that WIN money is for job search expenses), making salient the premises for being entitled to support, which in turn renders the client's actions as problematic. The client, however, does not acknowledge this, but instead justifies this faulty action on other grounds (i.e. concern for the children), thereby displaying that this transgression will be pursued knowingly and willingly (lines 6–7). This, in turn, makes the staff member respond by, on the one hand, picking up and drawing on the displayed concern for the children and, on the other, making the consequences for the same children salient to the client, if transgressing the activity-tied obligations (lines 8–9). When scrutinising how such indexical features are made relevant in interaction, the client and social worker constitute an interdependent and reciprocal category-pair (see Chapter 8 on resistance).

To follow up and report

Categorisation analysis may reveal how institutionally sanctioned work is being pursued in cases where clients resist participation in expected ways (see Chapter 8 on resistance). The social worker will find it difficult to fulfil the obligations of pursuing the case if the client does not cooperate. This is especially the case in the last example where a case of 'neglect' is discussed in a case conference in the UK.

Categorising reportable actions

The parents are not attending the case conference and the social worker (SW) gives her account of the current situation to her colleagues. In this extract a family support worker (CSW) and a nursery worker (SS) also join in and contribute to her account.

Extract 7 (from a corpus of data in Paula Doherty's doctoral project[1])

1	SW:	right, so we're here for the core group for [child] today. I went up today. Well
2		I was going up their street which is like the cresta run
3	CSW:	right
4	SW:	and I saw them coming down so they were half way up and I was half way
5		down. Err, so I stopped the car and put my handbrake on and jumped out and
6		said, are you coming to the core group. No, we didn't know it was on. So I
7		said, I told you, you've had a letter. I said, and I've also texted your three
8		different mobile phone numbers this morning and [mum] looked at [dad] and
9		[dad] said no, we're not coming. And I went, do you realise that obviously
10		now I'm reporting to court everything really. Err, no we're not coming, we're
11		going shopping.
12	CSW:	right
13	SW:	so I had a look at [child]. He was. He had a coat on and hat. But he didn't have
14		his mittens on. The mitten were in the pram, but obviously it was cold
15	SS:	minus eight wasn't it
16	SW:	I don't know where they were going to be honest. I said that I need to do CP
17		visits, but at present we've got a bit of a problem that they're disengaging
18		completely

([1]   The project is funded by a CASE Studentship Reference: ES/H028919/1.)

The social worker is reporting from her latest interaction with the parents. As we can note, it is not an ordinary report from a home visit, where certain observations of the child have been made and are being reported as instances of 'good' or 'bad' parenting. This account, in the form of a narrative, is re-enacting a recent event through reported speech (see Chapter 10 on reported speech). By animating the voice of herself and the father in a dialogue and by making the mother's non-verbal actions salient as actions in the unfolding event, she creates a common 'here and now' where the teller can make the listeners participate in a, for them, imagined event. As a result the 'disengagement' of the parents is not only described in general terms, but is actually enacted. As a result the transgression of the norms and expectations of these parents becomes salient. Under this kind of supervision, parents rather need to display 'concern' and 'engagement' to counteract being categorised as disengaged with their child. As can be noted, however, being disengaged with the case conference or the social worker herself is only one part of the story told. In addition, the observation of the child in the pram without 'his mittens on' (line 14) in the cold weather becomes another significant sign of neglect, in a history of reported observations.

As a teacher, police or health worker identifies concerns about a child, for example an injury or observation of parenting practices, they are obliged to contact the social services duty team. If the concerns are considered serious, the child may be removed from the family. More often the child remains at home and the social worker completes an assessment to determine if the child is at risk of 'significant harm'. In these cases it becomes quite clear that the professional also runs the risk of being reported for faulty action, if proper measures are not taken. The interdependency of the category-pair of the social worker and the client becomes even more salient as norms of conduct are violated or transgressed by one of the parties. Social workers' case documentation, police reports, teachers' accounts and personal stories from family members need to be assembled, to be worked up through par-ticular practices and meet the institutional criteria in order to be transformed into a 'child-at-risk' case. The 'social worker', the 'teacher' and the 'parent' also become institutionally interdependent in relation to the identification of 'a child at risk'. The categorisation of the case makes them institutionally accountable to varying degrees, in terms of not only what they cannot do but also what they can, should or must do in various situations (Hall *et al.* 2012).

Implications for social work practice

To make salient the implications of what has been earlier shown through examples from social work interaction, I will now reverse the picture. Even though we seem to have illuminated work at what is sometimes referred to as the 'micro level' – the everyday business of ordinary people talking to each other – we are at the core of what constitutes society. If you think of it, we are always in a situation, and this fact cannot be escaped. Talk and text in interaction is contextual and situated whatever, whenever and however we discuss matters, and regardless of whether we consider them to be of 'macro nature'. Debates and theories about social problems are largely negotiations precisely about how problems are to be understood. They include issues of how problems should be defined, how they should be empirically identified or observable, what should be done and who is responsible. These arguments always move between particular observations or examples as instances of, or deviations from, a set of available general categorisations.

As long as social issues have been formulated as problems and as tasks for governments to deal with, some categories have been central in the descriptions of problems as well as of targeted groups. These categories are, according to the philosopher Hacking (1986), generated from the ways of classifying that became necessary to deal with dilemmas in the context of the emerging bureaucracies and institutions of industrialised societies. As institutional categories they have long since been established and taken for granted as social facts, and have been followed up over time. Social problems (as well as targeted groups) are often represented in numerical form to get an overview, and to follow how the proportion of 'victims of abuse' or 'children at risk' change over time and how effective institutional measures are in managing them. But institutional categories such as these can never match reality no matter how sophisticated. They will inevitably shed light on some types of problems, while others fall in the shade. This also means that we can only learn about how they work by actually approaching the environments and actors who are directly involved and by studying their daily use in activities and interactions. Categorisations in social work practices are, as shown through these examples, interactively and discursively achieved, established and maintained. They make up the backbone of social work through talk and text practices. Such practices are necessary elements of everyday social work – they are built into institutional processes through encounters with clients, through meetings of different kinds and through electronic case notes and reports.

In social work interaction categories are consequential and have serious implications for the people concerned by providing access to or denial of services. An 'unemployed' person may, for instance, lose or receive benefits, or an 'elderly' person may be provided with or denied support to live at home. Categorisations in social work interaction also have a potential of shaping the identities of individuals, and may become either enabling or stigmatising. How will Robin cope, for example, if the description of him as being 'a very good liar' becomes salient in his relation to friends or significant adults in his life? And what will the future hold for Shane in terms of possibilities for intellectual stimulation once identified as having 'learning difficulties'? Such implications are most likely profound for young people's self-images and future possibilities. Also, the future identities of grown-ups might depend on whether they are identified as suitable or not, for instance to adopt a child or to take care of their own children. As Hacking (1986) argues, there is a risk that people come to fit their categories. To identify oneself as a 'disengaged parent' will most likely become a problem in its own right that adds to the difficulties of establishing faith in institutional interventions and in trusting the process of finding alternative ways to manage the situation (Hall *et al.* 2012).

However, social workers are also tied to the categorisations they pursue, and their legitimacy as 'social workers' depends on how they succeed in establishing and maintaining a trusting and productive relationship with clients. They are accountable in face-to-face situations, and through the observations and descriptions they make of clients for institutional purposes.

As institutional actors, they are also accountable to the public and politicians. The reports they write constitute an important basis by means of which we are informed about social problems and of how efficient institutional measures are to remedy them. These tensions and potential consequences of categorisation practices (for the clients on the one hand and the political and public on the other) create specific problems and dangers for social work. Measures that are politically targeted to specific groups, such as 'unemployed immigrants' or 'teenage mothers', often become paradoxical in their use. This is precisely because they are *targeted at a category* rather than at people and their concrete life situations and problems. These measures accordingly take a classification as their starting point. Since we know from empirical studies that, once established, categories tend to be taken for granted and are often transparent for the people who use them, this involves particular risks in social work practices. It is so easy to take a step further – that is, to search for and *ascribe to the individual person* the specific features of what was originally created as an institutional measure. This may result in acts of discrimination and is deeply problematic. By taking category analysis of interaction seriously, such acts of discrimination are possible to identify and scrutinise. There are examples of when people, as a consequence of being targeted in this manner, come to share a common history that enables them to explicitly resist being categorised accordingly, as in Juhila's study of shelter residents talking back (Juhila 2004).

When a category has been generated to serve as a tool for institutional purposes and interventions and is taken for granted, one should be aware that it may transform into a socially discriminating or stigmatising category. Categorisation in social work interaction is, however, a necessity and as a productive means it also provides possibilities for people involved to learn and to develop their capacities in managing their own lives. Scrutinising categorisation in social work interaction is a way to analyse and make visible many important features of social work practices. It offers opportunities to share and understand some features of everyday work that, on the one hand, are an evident part of everyday practice, but, on the other, are elusive and hard to notice in the ongoing interaction with clients.

4

ACCOUNTABILITY

Maureen Matarese and Dorte Caswell

```
1   CM:    you hear me? you have another-what's today, the fourth? You have another:
2          week (.) to get a TB and a psych in here (.) or else I'm going=
3   C:     =like I said Wednesday is my slowest day.
4   CM:    Wednesday I want you to be here at 1 o' clock, I don't want you to be even
5          working
6   C:     no no, I'll be here at 1 o' clock.
7   CM:    please (.) you need me to come here and I'll escort you over there so I can
8          ensure that you'll be it done? I need it done (.) I need to schedule you for it (.)
9          but you need to get it done (.) I need you to get a TB.
```

After several meetings between caseworker Innis and Michael, her client at the homeless shelter, he had still not completed the minimal tasks necessary for him to move forward. There was a mismatch between what was expected of him (that he complete those tasks) and his actions. His caseworker gives him an ultimatum with an incomplete threat, lest he continues to be non-compliant and to not attend meetings for his tuberculosis test and psychiatric evaluation in the next week (lines 1–2). The caseworker, in lines 7–9, concludes with a brief description of their individual responsibilities vis-à-vis these assigned tasks: she *schedules* him for tasks, and he *completes* those tasks by attending the necessary meetings. In fulfilling their individual responsibilities, both would maintain accountability.

Accountability and responsibility can be something that is talked *about*. By looking at *how* it is talked about, we can gain a richer understanding of how social work gets done and how accountability and responsibility get accomplished in social work contexts. For example, in the illustration above, the caseworker gives the client an ultimatum and begins a threat (line 2). In so doing, she is threatening her client's 'face', his desire to be liked.

She continues to apply pressure in line 4, where she stipulates that even his job should not prohibit him from attending the meeting. We can observe that there may be a gap between his *expectations* of pressure to attend meetings and the reality of that expressed pressure when talking with his caseworker. We stated earlier that, in lines 7–9, the caseworker defines their individual responsibilities at the shelter (a description of what is stated), but what discourse analysis shows us is that the description of responsibilities is also a justification that highlights the caseworker's *awareness* of the need to explain a potential mismatch between what her client expects from her and what she is actually doing. Her account provides justification for the pressure she is placing on him. The justification does double duty here: it wards off potential resistance from the client by explaining the caseworker's reasons for pressuring him, and it illustrates for us, the observers, that the caseworker deemed that amount of pressure worthy of discursive backup – suggesting that perhaps less pressure or pressure less forcefully delivered may not necessarily have warranted a justification. From this illustration, then, we learn that accountability can be both a topic (X client must do Y task in order to be a responsible client) and a discursive device for managing untoward, unexpected behaviour (Scott and Lyman 1968; Mäkitalo 2003). Lipsky (1980) suggests that social workers are held accountable by their administration as well as by their clients who request or demand action from them. Social workers are often asked to account for the behaviour of their clients as well as account for their own actions as professionals, and clients are also held accountable in their meetings with social workers. Accountability, therefore, operates across the social work professional spectrum and is not unidirectional.

Traditionally, accountability has been discussed at length in literature and research on new public management, or rather not-so-new public management (Hanlon and Rosenberg 1998). This has also been referred to as new managerialism, which in part suggests that, as social institutions are increasingly treated like businesses, accountability measures have become more stringent (Banks 2004). While accountability is often understood in this policy-level, top-down kind of way, we suggest that perhaps the concept should also be approached from a bottom-up, discourse perspective.

We will argue that the concept of accountability needs more detailed attention on a micro-analytic level. In so doing, we may understand not only whether accountability is an issue in social work (or not) but *how* accountability is achieved in everyday social work and to what ends. A discourse analytic perspective highlights the small, nuanced ways in which accountability is constructed, negotiated and achieved, allowing us to see that accountability is happening not just when managerial oversight is involved or when the topic is about client responsibility. It also occurs in small ways during everyday meetings between social workers and clients or between social workers and supervisors.

Through this chapter we illustrate the small micro instances of account-ability that occur in everyday social work and that colour the broader understandings of the concept. By looking at social worker interactions in two institutionally similar contexts in two different countries, we describe how accountability works on an interactional level with different sets of par-ticipants, as well as how some accounts are coloured with moral judgements and others are not.

Theoretical background

The literature on accounts is broad and encompasses numerous different perspectives and research traditions. In their overview of accounts, Potter and Wetherell (1987) compare the treatment of accounts in social psychol-ogy studies as well as in conversation analysis. They argue that, while the former tradition has primarily been focused on *types* of accounts, the latter has been focused on accounts as conversational acts positioned in sequences of talk. We follow this latter approach, the basis for which begins with Garfinkel's (1967) ethnomethodology: the study of structural properties of mundane, everyday actions and expressions. Garfinkel expressly describes the importance of studying accounts and accountability, which are elicited and accomplished in everyday, seemingly uninteresting moments. This chapter focuses on the way in which accountability is talked into being and negotiated through everyday social work talk.

Accountability in social interaction

Goffman (1959) was perhaps the first to note the importance of accounts in institutional contexts in his analysis of institutional encounters and processes. Accounts are common responses to questions prompting an explanation. They constitute important narratives that are variable as well as interested and constructive (Antaki 1994). Buttny and Morris (2001: 285–286) point out a number of directions, such as 'accounts as recon-figuring the context of an event, accounts as reality negotiation, accounts as narratives, accounts as an exception to the rule, accounts as a dispre-ferred response and so on'. However, the most common distinction is one between accounts *for* actions (answering for troublesome behaviour) and accounts *of* actions (descriptions or narratives of events), the former of which is addressed in this chapter. The chapter devoted to narrative (Chapter 6) addresses the latter type of account.

Scott and Lyman's (1968) foundational paper explores the accounts of actions in detail, arguing that verbal accounts help to explain unanticipated or untoward behaviour, 'bridg[ing] the gap between action and expectation . . . throw[ing] bridges between the promised and the performed' (1968: 46).

Accounts, according to Scott and Lyman, can have a mitigating, softening, or 'neutralising' function (1968: 46). The study of deviance and the study of accounts are intertwined, as accounts are often called upon to clarify deviant behaviour. The two most common types of accounts described in the literature are *excuses* and *justifications*, initially addressed by Austin (1962). Excuses admit the (potentially offensive) act, but ultimately deny responsibility, often displacing blame (e.g. 'I know I was late, but the subway was behind schedule'). Justifications, on the other hand, generally accept responsibility but provide alternate views of the act (e.g. 'While I did forget to clean under the bed no one really looks under there anyway, right?'). Scott and Lyman (1968) also discuss a related concept, *scapegoating*, which locates responsibility in another situation or person. Examples of scapegoating are seen in several extracts in this chapter.

Scott and Lyman (1968) identify a number of different accounting styles that range in degrees of social intimacy, only one of which is relevant in this chapter: the *consultative* style. This style is used when one interlocutor is seeking information/knowledge from another. Often requests for background information are made, and accounts are thorough and detailed, in comparison to the short in-group minimal responses in intimate and casual accounts. The consultative style appears to emphasise a knowledge imbalance between participants, in which one participant is seeking knowledge or information from another. This power imbalance among participants is reflected in our data, as it is for most institutional talk (Drew and Heritage 1992b). This chapter, therefore, deals specifically with differing types of consultative accounts, including justifications and excuses.

Accounts: responsibility and moral categorisation in social work

Juhila *et al.* (2010: 76) suggest that 'accounting is an inherent part of all human service practices as it is part of social interaction in general'. It is, therefore, an appropriate and necessary subject of study for social work research. Accountability and responsibility are inherently tied, particularly in institutional settings. Mäkitalo (2003: 496) argues that 'being responsible in institutional encounters thus implies being able to respond in accountable and comprehensible manners as we engage in them'. Accounting, therefore, highlights how we do responsibility and how we take responsible action. It explores the taking of responsible action in different contexts, including how spouses shift positions regarding their responsibilities in couples therapy sessions (Kurri and Wahlström 2005), how moral categories of responsibility are constructed in child protection contexts (Hall *et al.* 2006), and how blame and excuses function vis-à-vis the presumption of responsible action in a supportive housing unit (Juhila and Raitakari 2010), to name only a few.

While some accounts address a lack of comprehensibility, others fall into a different category of moral accounts: accounts that position participants according to moral categories. As such, *moral categorisation* has become increasingly relevant in accountability literature, particularly in social work contexts. Hall *et al.* (2006) suggest that accounts can reveal the ways in which participants position themselves and others vis-à-vis moral categories. Juhila (2003), for example, describes the moral positioning of 'good' vs. 'bad' clients, 'bad' parent etc. In this book, Chapter 3 on categorisation has a substantive review of that perspective. The construction and positioning of others according to moral categories is a common by-product of accounts, particularly when the account is managing a transgression or a gap between expectation and action (Scott and Lyman 1968). There are a variety of factors that shape accounts, including attention to face wants (Goffman 1967), preference structure (Silverman 1997) and various features of politeness (Brown and Levinson 1978), which can soften or mitigate accusations/ elicitations and accounts. Preference structure and the management of face wants in justifications and excuses are particularly addressed in the empirical portion of this chapter.

In sum, then, the interactions we present in this chapter bring to light various shades of accounts. Our main focus will be on justifications and excuses, as they occur in seemingly mundane social work interaction. These accounts include differing levels of threats to face and moral categorisation and each highlights the way in which gaps between expectation and action are managed between participants. We look at accounts as devices and show how it is possible to make them visible through analysis of social work interaction.

Accounts and accountability in social work interaction: data examples and analyses

The following extracts present five different illustrations of accounts in social work interaction. They vary in participant type (supervisor and social worker, social worker and client etc.), as well as in the type of account being used. While most involve justifications, and are in the consultative style (Scott and Lyman 1968), the way in which the justifications are elicited and managed varies. Some empirical examples represent different levels of conflict or potential conflict between the different participants in social work interaction. The cases are drawn from two distinctly different national contexts (American and Danish) and from social work interactions within the area of unemployment as well as homelessness. Drawing on the literature above, we use discourse analysis that draws from conversation analysis (Drew and Heritage 1992b; Sacks 1992), in addition to the literature described above.

Extended account by a social worker for justifying service needs

The first case is from an interaction between a social worker from a Danish Job Centre (SW), one social worker from an activation measure called 'Handy Job' (HD) and the client Tobias (C). The social workers at the Job Centre have an institutional task of implementing active labour market measures for the unemployed. Especially towards the under 25 year old, this is an essential part of policy, and thus an important institutional task for the social worker. Handy Job is one of a number of activation measures in the municipality. Present at the meeting is also another social worker from the activation measure as well as a researcher, neither of whom contribute in the extract below. The client is a young man who has recently turned 18. He is diagnosed with Asperger's syndrome. The extract is from the very start of the interaction, in which the social worker from the Job Centre introduces the client to the other social workers. The extract is interesting because of the social worker's extensive account in which he tries to justify why the meeting has been arranged. This first extract reveals an account for a future action (Buttny and Morris 2001), which highlights the gap between expectation (that Tobias should participate in Handy Job) and action (that Tobias may not fit the client profile for Handy Job). Here, the social worker from the Job Centre (SW) provides a lengthy justification sequence that explains why services are needed for the client, Tobias.

Extract 1

1	SW:	what I can <u>briefly</u> say is that it is <u>me</u> who has established the contact to this place or have
2		asked for this meeting (.)
3	HD:	°yes°
4	SW:	and that is simply because (.) Tobias is receiving a cash benefit right now
5	HD:	[yes]
6	SW:	[and] he wants to move on with his life and would like to get a job (1) and that is sort of
7		(1) what we in one way or another (1) need to help him with (.) and there is <u>also</u> the issue
8		it is (1) that (1) you have a diagnosis
9	C:	yes Asperger [syndrome]
10	SW:	[Asperger] and that is why (.) it is not <u>only</u> just employment (.) which
11		needs to be in focus
12	HD:	°no°
13	SW:	there are <u>also</u> some other issues that need to be in focus right now amongst other things (.)
14		you need structure and need someone who sort of <u>holds you on</u> track if you have some
15		bad periods you have expressed this yourself right and you can explain this in greater
16		detail (1) we have been to different places (.) we have been to the school of production
17		and we have been to ((name of activation offer)) to look at some stuff and then we have
18		<u>chosen</u> to say anyway okay now we will have a look at 'Handy Job' before

19			[we talk about
20	HD:		[yes hmm
21	SW:	what <u>will be</u> the <u>best</u> place for Tobias and what the best offer will be (2) and I have to say
22		again that in the long run possibly I will not be the caseworker but I want to because
23		typically Asperger is not in the Job Centre
24	HD:	no
25	SW:	but I would like to present the case now while I've got it (.) move on so that we can move
26		on with Tobias
27	HD:	yes okay
28	SW:	so the purpose is that (.) you explain a bit about what <u>you</u> (.) sort of (.) would (.) like to do
29		and the you ((addressed at the other social workers)) explain what you sort of can offer
30		and then we will have to talk about what we evaluate if Tobias is the target group for this
31		[place]
32	HD:	[yes]
33	SW:	because that is important or if you think that maybe he belongs to a different place

This extract illustrates a lengthy, but successful justification sequence in which there is no orientation by any participant to interactional trouble. It begins with the pre-sequence 'what I can briefly say', which prepares HD for the coming justification. Extract 1 reveals several discursive practices that together make this justification hold water for HD. This extract illustrates a situation in which the social worker claims authority and provides a detailed and satisfactory account to HD. The social worker introduces the account through a pre-sequence, which justifies the reason for the meeting while also establishing epistemic authority through words such as 'me', which the SW emphasises intonationally (line 1). The pre-sequence also claims the floor, which he holds by using continuers such as 'and' at the beginning of each new utterance. HD's only contributions tend to be backchannel devices that allow SW to maintain the floor, such as 'yes' in lines 3 and 5. The SW's turns are lengthy and include specific details about the client's situation.

In this extract, there are several efforts at mitigation, which appear to be used in order to displace blame from SW. Words such as 'briefly' respect negative politeness, appealing to one's desire to not be bothered (Brown and Levinson 1978), and 'simply' (line 4) downgrades the situation, making it appear less severe. His use of passive voice ('it is me who has established the contact' – lines 1–2) also functions to distance him from associated blame for calling a meeting in the first place (as no one likes meetings, period). The social worker then explains that Tobias, who is present, is receiving a cash benefit, and he constructs him as a responsible, 'good client' (Juhila 2003). This is done through a moral categorisation of him as one who seeks to move forward but who also has a psychiatric diagnosis, Asperger's syndrome – a complicating factor. He constructs Tobias's trouble through softening devices. This is done using ambiguous terminology such as 'other issues', 'other things' and 'stuff', all of which define the type of job he is applying for. SW continues to hedge, suggesting that he might not be his caseworker for long (lines 22–23), and characterises himself as going out of his way (lines 25–26) to help Tobias when he does not need to, thereby categorising himself as a 'good' social worker who has the moral high ground; however, it also serves as an excuse should this client not do what he is supposed to do. If Tobias is not part of the caseworker's load, then he cannot claim responsibility for what happens to him in the future.

He shifts between aligning himself with Tobias and talking among the professionals. He refers to a lot of different institutional framings of the interaction and the options for action including his own responsibilities as a social worker. The social worker establishes alignment and empathy with HD, using 'you', which, while talking about Tobias's needs, positions HD as a recipient in need as well. Moreover, the worker's use of 'we' refers to his work with the client, highlighting the tasks he and the client have completed collaboratively.

This first extract provides an example of accounting that justifies particular actions and, while the account is lengthy, what we see here is the way in which the social worker holds the floor (using pre-sequences and 'and'), establishes himself as credible (epistemic authority) and successfully informs HD of the situation without any real trouble occurring. This account is accomplished in collaboration with the other participants in the meeting; however, in some cases the accomplishment of an account takes far more work. The following extract reveals one such instance, in which a supervisor does not find the account of the social worker adequate. The supervisor's responses to the social worker signal interactional trouble.

Supervisor prompts an account from a social worker

Our second case is drawn from a regular team meeting in the cash benefit department within a Danish Job Centre. Six social workers and a supervisor are present along with a researcher who observes the interaction. Social worker A (SWa) presents a case of a young man who has previously been a cash benefit recipient. He has made numerous attempts at an apprenticeship, but he has failed to finish every time. SWa wants acceptance from the supervisor to grant the client two hours of weekly support from a mentor. They talk back and forth about the history of the client, his family background and his possible lack of social competences. In this extract the supervisor has a face-threatening turn, to which the social worker promptly reacts by giving an account. The case is interesting because the presentation of the client abruptly goes from someone who has had trouble getting into the labour market, partly due to outside factors (such as starting an apprenticeship in a company with a bad track record of handling apprentices poorly), to someone who has vast and serious social and other problems.

Extract 2

1	SWa:	<u>no</u> he was not a drug [abuser]
2	SWb:	[really]
3	SWa:	or he is not abusing and the mentor (2) <u>has</u> (2) sort of (2) tried to (1)
4		get him (2) to understand (.) what it means to (1) be in a work place and
5		that sort of thing but there is <u>nothing</u> else to do than to just <u>try</u> it, and
6		then say oh well that is what we do
7	Sup:	but the mentor he had in his <u>ordinary</u> apprenticeship was that
8		a mentor who was brought in from <u>outside</u> or someone
9		at the work place?
10	SWa:	it was someone from the work place
11	Sup:	[okay]
12	SWa:	[I] <u>think</u> it was (3) him (2) the grocer himself
13	Sup:	okay
14	SWa:	°yes°
15	Sup:	yes (2) okay (2)
16	SWc:	but they don't [treat their employees]
17	Sup:	[no I was just] about to say if it had been an
18		<u>external</u> consultant the he possibly could have nipped it in the bud
19	SWc:	[yes]
20	Sup:	[but] if it was someone from the inside then it is easier to understand isn't it?
21	SWc:	yes
22	Sup:	but what <u>is it</u> he can't do that he needs a mentor for? I still need to get that
23		illuminated
24	SWa:	well he is (.) a former abuser (1) he has <u>anxiety</u> and <u>social phobia</u> (.) he has a
25		<u>depression</u> (2) yes (.) <u>and</u> then he has all these (.) or he <u>doesn't</u> have these (.)
26		social competences

Extract 2 is more clearly a justification that highlights the gap opened through a transgression, wherein expectation (that the social worker should make clear why the client needs the mentor) and subsequent action (that the social worker fails to do so) do not overlap. Preference structure, then, reveals this gap, as the information provided by the social worker continually falls short of the supervisor's expectations. SWa's assertion that the client is 'not a drug abuser' is called into question by SWb, whose 'really' prompts clarification. SWa orients to SWb's statement as a clarification request by equivocating and clarifying using 'or' and providing an extended description of the client's status. The social worker downgrades the extent to which she really tried to help the client understand (lines 3–4). The word 'tried' generally implies a (partially or entirely) failed attempt; with the downgrade 'sort of', it is unclear how much the mentor really did.

The supervisor, however, treats SWa's clarification as persistently inadequate. Her presumed expectation is that SWa explains why the client requires a mentor, explanations that have yet to be satisfactory. The supervisor establishes disagreement through 'but' and a follow-up question (lines 7–9). The supervisor merely confirms receipt of that information while presumably waiting for her to satisfy the need for a richer account of why a mentor is needed for this client. SWa's clarification is still deemed inadequate given the supervisor's 'okay', which signals a desire for SWa to continue holding the floor. Likewise, SWa's answer (line 10) calls into question her epistemic authority ('I think'). A second prompt for the social worker to continue (line 13) is acknowledged by SWc who begins to clarify. The brief sub-conversation between SWc and the supervisor concludes with the supervisor reorienting to SWa and directly asking why the client requires a mentor, a noteworthy request given SWa's discursive work in establishing the client's needs thus far. The questioning of this basic issue by the supervisor (lines 21–22) and the request for clarification make this turn quite face-threatening. The supervisor calls on the social worker to 'illuminate', or prove, the need for a mentor. Pushed in this regard, SWa provides an account, or justification, for the use of a mentor. In so doing, she morally categorises the client as deviant (abuser, anxiety, social phobia, depression) in order to justify her decision to use a mentor, and deviant moral categories often highlight failures in accountability (Juhila 2003). SWa uses 'yes' (line 25) to verbally confirm that her assessment is legitimate.

In this extract, then, the supervisor elicits an account that justifies the practitioner's behaviour; however, these small, overt moments do not sufficiently address how accountability is constructed in social work interaction. In fact, even this example of an account includes other related practices (moral categorisation etc.). In everyday social work practice, accountability may be constructed using accounts but also a repertoire of other discursive practices.

In acknowledging her lack of understanding regarding the mentor, the supervisor signals interactional trouble. As such, perhaps this counts as a request for an account for actions (Buttny and Morris 2001). More importantly, this extract serves as an example of a prompt for a verbal account. SWa begins with discourse marker 'well', which suggests disagreement and hesitation, before providing a laundry list of client diagnoses that establish his need for mentoring, satisfying the supervisor's request. Paradoxically, this turns out later in the interaction to be endangering the granting of a mentor, as this causes the supervisor to question if this is really the right measure for a client with such severe problems.

The extract highlights the supervisor's pursuit of a satisfactory account from the social worker, as well as the interactional work that needs to be done in order to elicit the needed answer. Backchannelling (e.g. mm-hmm, uh-huh), while often signalling affiliation, here appears to acknowledge interactional trouble, given SWa's subsequent unsatisfactory responses. This trouble is only alleviated when the needed information is provided. It is possible that such persistence by the supervisor could be viewed as accumulating threats to the social worker's face and epistemic authority. Importantly, then, attending to accounting practices does not simply mean attending to the individual *doing* the accounting but also to the elicitation of the account. How might the supervisor have elicited more detailed information more quickly, for example?

Caseworker eliciting an account from her client

The next extract illustrates a different sort of account – one in which a shelter caseworker elicits an account from a client after a morally loaded threat to his face. This case is from a caseworker–client interaction in a New York City homeless shelter. In this meeting, the caseworker (CM) and the client (C) were discussing his employment, a prerequisite for acquiring housing options, when she threatens his face with an accusation, causing the need for a justification account.

Extract 3

1	C:	I'll be getting me a job, already got a job, I told 'em that
2		but they just one –
3	CM:	where's your job at?
4	C:	out in college point, for XXX.
5	CM:	that's not gonna work. so here's=
6	C:	=what do I do?
7	CM:	you need to comply with them.
8	C:	I AM COMPLYING WITH THEM I WAS GOING TO THE PROGRAM THING
9		EVERYDAY AND WHEN
10		I WAS GOING THEY DON'T WANNA HEAR THAT!
11		((yelling))
12	CM:	I'm talking about now cause we remember we had to do your case all over
13		again, so now your case is open, right?

This extract occurs towards the beginning of a meeting and is yet another one that signals interactional trouble. In this meeting, the client mentions that he will be getting (or has already got) a job. When the caseworker presses the client on the location of the job, and the distance is deemed too far by the caseworker, she begins to provide an alternate approach ('so here's'). The client interrupts his caseworker with a follow-up question. The caseworker, in line 7, uses the personal pronoun 'you'. This can be seen as a device to attribute responsibility and obligation to the client in conjunction with deontic modal 'need' (Coates 1983). Her statement, however, is ultimately face-threatening, implying that he has not yet complied with the Job Centre that provides public assistance funds. Her utterance 'you need to comply with them' is constructed in such a way as to accuse him of currently being in a state of non-compliance, signalling interactional trouble. In so doing, the caseworker positions him as a 'bad client' (Juhila 2003), an orientation that is confirmed by how the client orients to her utterance: through a justification that denies the offence entirely and provides a scapegoat (Scott and Lyman 1968). His response (lines 8–10) distances him from the transgression, and his shouting/raised voice indexes his awareness of trouble. The client rebuts her challenge by using her language ('comply with them') and then accounts for his actions in the public assistance programme. His justification prompts an account from his caseworker (lines 12–13) as well.

Here, then, we see that accounts can be successfully accomplished between social workers, and between social workers and their supervisors (as seen in Extracts 1 and 2), as well as by clients when requested by the worker. This extract is probably the most obvious type of account, particularly in consultative contexts (Scott and Lyman 1968) in which the client is applying to the caseworker for help; the inherent asymmetry would position the client as needing to provide justification to his caseworker. However, as Lipsky (1980) suggests, social workers are also held accountable by their clients, as shown in the next extract.

Client tries to elicit an account from a caseworker

Extract 4 takes place in the same context as the prior example, although with different participants. Here, a shelter caseworker enquires about her homeless client's completion of a task, and he accuses her of having never given him an appointment for the meeting. This caseworker and client had met several times before. In this interaction the caseworker is enquiring as to whether her client, Michael, received his psychiatric evaluation, a requirement for all clients at the shelter.

Extract 4

1	CM:	((question: too quiet to hear. She enquires about his completion of his psychiatric
2		evaluation?))
3	C:	no cause you never gave me the appointment
4	CM:	Michael, you know your psych evaluation was for Friday, I was busy
5	C:	yeah but I need a paper to come here or else they ain't gonna
6		attend me
7	CM:	did you try to see me on Friday?

In this extract, the account is yet again a signal of interactional trouble. The client levels an accusation at his caseworker, a face-threatening move that highlights the gap between expectation and action; this time the expectations are both the client's and the caseworker's. The first mismatch between expectation (getting the evaluation) and action (not getting the evaluation) is identified by the client through his accusation. However, his accusation (line 3) identifies yet another gap – between his expectations of her assistance and her actions (not providing an appointment slip). This second account is managed and addressed by the caseworker through her justification for her transgression (line 4). The caseworker uses the client's prior knowledge as a scapegoat (Scott and Lyman 1968) for her unanticipated action, distancing her from his accusation by resting ultimate responsibility with him (line 4). She additionally provides an excuse that admits the transgression but offers some extenuating circumstances that serve to legitimise it (Buttny 1993). Her offer of an excuse justifies her transgression, suggesting that she was busy. This extract, like the one earlier, refers to some transgression prior to the account that includes moral categorisation. As with 'you did not comply' (Extract 3) and 'you never gave me the appointment' (Extract 4), this is a moral categorisation. However, in this case the client is categorising or positioning the caseworker as 'not doing case/social work'. She is positioned as deficient in completing her professional duties.

Her justification is dispreferred and not accepted by the client, who once again challenges her by foisting responsibility back on his caseworker through a scapegoat tactic (lines 5–6). In line 7, the caseworker places ultimate responsibility back with the client who did not request proper paperwork at her office. This extract highlights the kind of management of justifications that can occur when the transgression (and the agent of the transgression) is not agreed upon. Neither party wanting to take blame or being willing to be morally categorised, accusations and moral categories are constructed and negotiated as they bid for a claim to be excused from blame.

These last few extracts involving interactional trouble of one sort or another (2–4) may be contrasted with the lengthier justification in Extract 1, in which the social worker accounts for certain treatment for a client. While interactional trouble is identified in Extract 3, the social worker is not being morally judged for a transgression. Instead, she morally categorises the client for his non-compliance. Extract 4, in contrast, highlights that accounts for transgressions can really work in either/both direction(s). These extracts, then, highlight that accounts and accountability are discursive practices that happen in everyday institutional talk and that may or may not involve the justification for morally loaded transgressions.

Accountability and accounting

Our last extract emphasises how several types of accountability may be happening at once. Here, we have a shelter caseworker accounting for a decision she has made about a client. Simultaneously, we see the ways accountability policy (macro-accountability) vis-à-vis the institution and city government circulates through and helps support the micro-level accounts the social worker is making to her client.

Extract 5

1	CM:	. . . the list (.) <u>see this list? you're on it</u> (.) you have to go (.)
2		Julio all these people highlighted have been here over 360 days (.) as
3		per ((shelter policy)) everyone who has been here for year
4		or more needs to <u>go</u> (.)
5		no you have to pick a <u>place</u> (.)
6	C:	what do you mean pick?
7	CM:	<u>you have to take a room</u> (.) <u>you have to take a room</u> (.) this
8		Thursday (.) don't miss it the 16th (.) see it? ((points to a calendar)) (.)
9		August 16th (.)
10	C:	Thursday?
11	CM:	clients that's been in the shelter too many days (,) you've been
12		here <u>417 days</u> (.) they want you outta here (.) you've been in at X
13		shelter (.) it's a lot of days to be in shelter (.) they want you out (.) so
14		I have to get the <u>brunt</u> of this (.)

In this final example, accountability as a thematic topic (rather than as a discourse feature per se) overlaps with the micro-level accounts that we have discussed thus far. This is one example of the top-down kind of accountability often discussed in social work literature merging with the bottom-up approach to accountability we have been focusing on in this chapter. In line 1, the caseworker (CM) tells her client (C) that he must leave the shelter. She then provides him with an extended account – a justification – that, like Extract 2, must be expanded upon due to interactional trouble. The first justification sequence (lines 2–4) begins with a reference to a shelter-wide memo that includes a list of highlighted names for clients who were in the shelter for 360 days or more and who therefore have priority for housing placement. She uses the homeless services policy to justify the pressure she is placing on him to leave (line 3). Again, the scapegoat approach to justifications is used here: both the policy and the city homeless services organisation are used as scapegoats that substantiate the pressure she places on the client.

The client, however, has limited English-speaking fluency, and therefore uses his turns to pose clarification questions. These can be identified as dispreferred responses, because they prompt the caseworker to provide additional information and clarification. She, therefore, renews her request that he leave the shelter (lines 6–7), and she provides yet another justification accounting for her request (lines 11–13). Her account begins with a general-ised subject, 'clients', distancing and depersonalising the policy from the client. Her subsequent statement, however, applies this rule to this particular client, citing the number of days he has lived in the shelter. By using 'they', the caseworker distances herself from decision making, explaining that the administration and city want him out of the shelter, given the length of time he has lived there (line 12). In the end, she involves him in understanding the pressure she is receiving ('getting the brunt of this') from the admin-istration, again distancing herself from responsibility by asking him to find housing and leave the shelter, and emphasising a higher authority as the ultimate scapegoat. This is also an example of how social workers are held accountable for client behaviour, as mentioned in the introduction, although it should be noted that other examples of accountability exist across many of the extracts provided in this book, particularly in Chapter 8 on resistance. The lenses and approaches described in this book (accountability, resistance, categorisation, delicacy etc.) do not occur in a vacuum. Instead, we spotlight each one individually to draw attention to the nuances of each, although in most cases one or more of these will occur in proximity to or simultaneously with others.

Implications for social work practice

Accountability evidences itself in large-scale policy initiatives and in the briefest sequences of talk. We have spent the majority of the chapter describing what we might call small 'a' accountability – everyday accounts that are talked into being through mundane social work interactions. However, as we have illustrated, several excerpts highlight larger, broader understandings of accountability within the interaction. Though certainly in other extracts, larger, policy-oriented notions of accountability were invoked most explicitly in Extract 5. Still, Extract 2 describes who qualifies for a mentor, which is a policy issue requiring responsible action. More-over, the caseworker's reference to compliance in Extract 3 and the client's insistence on having proper paperwork in Extract 4 both speak to more macro senses of accountability.

Accountability on a policy or administrative level is often discussed in social work coursework and textbooks. It undergirds social work policy and finds its way into practice. Since the 1980s, new managerialist approaches have been integrated into social and human service institutions and, often with a neoliberal philosophical approach, create social institutions that resemble business institutions in their structure and organisation. New managerialism utilises bureaucratic, management-oriented organisational structures to improve the functioning and efficiency of social institutions. While many competing ideologies function in social institutions, neoliberal approaches to social/human services have been widely acknowledged and critiqued (Fairclough 2000; Harlow 2003; Taylor 2003). As this approach has impacted social work, service delivery has also been affected. Paperwork practices instituted as part of increasing accountability standards have reconstructed practice such that client narratives are reduced (White *et al.* 2009). Interactions with clients are constrained, moreover, by the organisation of required documents and computer-mediated forms, which present series of questions and topics to be covered and recorded.

Social workers who are now part of this new paradigm need to be aware of the tenets of the practice vis-à-vis the constraints placed on those practices by institutions, policies and other governing bodies. 'New accountability', which describes increasing accountability requirements within modern management, establishes a tension between professional practices established by the field and accountability practices established by the organisation/ institution, posing a threat to professional ethics (Banks 2004). Though not in discourse analysis, Banks (2004: 150) suggests that:

> To be accountable is literally to be liable to be called upon to give an account of what one has done or not done. The account may include all or some of descriptions, explanations, excuses or justifications. Frequently giving an account is associated with the occurrence of a problematic situation and the apportioning of blame.

Lipsky (1980) suggests that accountability systems implemented across social institutions structure institutional practices in ways that counter the original intentions of the disciplines. The practitioner, moreover, who Lipsky calls a 'street-level bureaucrat', puts policy into practice in their everyday work and mediates between the administration and the client. The practitioner must hold clients accountable and be held accountable themselves by their administration. These accountability systems shift some traditionally communicative facets of social work into people processing, and various strategies have been developed to deal with the tension between the individualised practices that social work promotes as a field and the uniform treatment of clients that is implicitly endorsed through this accountability system. Although Lipsky is famous for his argument that policy is ultimately created by street-level bureaucrats, such as social workers rather than politicians, recent research in social work argues that, due to new models of accountability and managerialism, the coping mechanisms used at the front line have changed substantially (Høybye-Mortensen 2013), possibly altering the conclusions of front-line bureaucracy research altogether.

A bottom-up perspective for the study of accountability in interactions, taking place at the very front line of social work, enables us to study the specific ways in which accounts are used and produced. It also enables us to see the multidimensional character of accountability. It is not purely something imposed on social workers from above, either from the institution or from the policy level, but surfaces in everyday social work interactions as well. While the managerial perspective on accountability is able to shed critical light on some aspects of social work, the micro-analytical perspective provides us with insights into the variety of devises used to *do* accountability every day.

Our data highlight how accountability is constructed through a variety of discourse practices including moral categorisation, role set definition/boundary work, deontic modals and deictic pronouns. Accountability is established through the definition of my work in relation to yours.

While many chapters in this book have direct implications for social workers (e.g. Chapter 9), where the discourse practices directly influence the delivery of social work values and concepts, accountability has a less direct but no less important impact. Systems of accountability surface through, shape and are shaped by social work practices. In some ways, accountability has always been present in social work, as practitioners have held their clients accountable for certain tasks and the social workers have been obliged to account for their time at work to their superiors. However, given the increase in accountability standards, and the means by which those standards are logged and verified, accountability is even more present in everyday, mundane social work interaction than in the past. A tension exists between what the field of social work asks of their practitioners and the bureaucratic necessities that seem peripherally relevant, but are no less present.

The way in which larger notions of accountability manifest themselves in the everyday practice of social workers, particularly through accounts, is vitally important to understand the daily influence of policy on practice. Attention to everyday manifestations of accountability, notwithstanding attention to larger policies, provides a lens through which social workers may understand the forms of talk that make up the fabric of their everyday work.

5

BOUNDARY WORK

Stef Slembrouck and Christopher Hall

Unlike other analytical concepts discussed in this book, boundary work is not essentially a concept associated with the analysis of discourse or interaction. Boundaries more generally have been the focus of much investigation. Tilly (2004: 213), for example, notes that:

> People everywhere organize a significant part of their social interaction around the formation, transformation, activation, and suppression of social boundaries. It happens at the small scale of interpersonal dialogue, at the medium scale of rivalry within organizations, and at the large scale of genocide. Us–them boundaries matter.

In the professional literature, the boundaries of work are seen in guidelines, expectations and rules that set ethical and technical standards, with discussions concentrating on potential problems and how these are to be contained. Boundaries 'set limits for safe, acceptable and effective behaviour by workers' (Cooper 2012: 11). These can be serious issues that could form the basis for disciplinary proceedings, for example abusive relations with clients, or matters of good practice, such as whether to lend money to a client (Reamer 2003) or how to deal with social situations in which neighbours turn out to be clients (Pugh 2007). Cooper (2012: 12) also notes how professional boundaries are not the same as the boundary rules of the workplace. However, dilemmas about what is or is not appropriate action in social work is a daily issue, not only from an ethical or organisational perspective, but also in terms of deciding on practical aspects of work, for example how much time to spend talking to the child and to the parent. As a family support worker notes:

FS: and so every week we would do 20 minutes' work with the child and then deconstruct it with the parent and think about what was going to happen next week, so some other parents would perhaps have seen a much more structured session out of that, but you find when the parents had more emotional needs themselves it was that kind of two sessions where some sessions would be about the child and some sessions would be more about the parent, and this is a parent that fell into that category.

For social workers, then, boundaries involve decision making about a wide range of matters concerning how to manage the detail of their encounters with clients.

As the application of guidelines and expectations inevitably comes with constraints and restrictions, the coercive and potentially conflictive dimensions of crossing boundaries must be raised too, and, with this, that of work *on* the boundaries. What are the implications of professionals crossing a boundary – whether sanctioned negatively as not permissible or assessed positively as going the extra mile (Doel *et al.* 2010: 1884), the possibility of clients resisting boundaries, or the occurrence of boundary work towards overcoming frontier and division?

To draw a boundary is both to enable cooperation within the constraints of a particular understanding and to exclude what is beyond the boundary. While the dynamics of boundaries in the production of social space, and of activities on or around the boundaries, have received much attention in social and cultural geography (de Certeau 1984; Lefebvre 1991), an obvious chord is struck with the kind of balancing activity that much of social work appears to revolve around: anything can be talked about *versus* a specific interventional remit informs the home visit; being supportive *versus* being directive; 'I help you with this' *versus* 'you take care of that'.

Boundary work

We refer to boundary work in this chapter as the ways in which social workers and clients manage the dilemmas of the personal, professional, organisational and cultural divisions during everyday encounters. More usually boundary work has been seen as the ways in which professionals seek to establish their skills and jurisdiction over a particular domain of work – what are sometimes called 'turf wars'. Gieryn (1983) first coined the term 'boundary work' to denote how scientists distinguish their work from that of non-science. Much of this literature is oriented to the ways in which professional workers negotiate and dispute boundaries between one another, defining certain tasks as (in)appropriate, or to how they harbour ambitions for increased rewards and status by taking on new tasks (Allen 2000). Boundaries are intrinsic to organisations and are reproduced in interaction

(Hernes 2004). There is no central stabilising function but a series of 'turf wars' – struggles for territory, professional or occupational rights and control (Allen 2000). Examples of such research include: how dieticians aim to increase their power and influence by establishing a 'vocabulary of their unique competence' (Wikström 2008: 68); how unqualified health care assistants take on tasks previously performed by other professionals (Nancarrow and Borthwick 2005: 898); and how members of the cardiology team promote their particular contributions in terms of expertise, competence and patient centredness (Sanders and Harrison 2008). Of particular interest is how 'new' professions struggle to identify a place for their skills in between traditional occupational groups (Sanders and Harrison 2008: 305), alongside evolving claims that appeal to an intra-professional value base. As an example of the latter, O'Leary *et al.* (2012: 3–4) note how social work's boundaries have been historically influenced by other professions in subscribing to a more traditional model of professional distance and separation from the client. In contrast, the authors advocate that 'whilst the ability to forge good interpersonal relationships is desirable, but often not essential for highly developed professions such as medicine and law, it is an absolute precondition of effective social work practice' (O'Leary *et al.* 2012: 3–4). Their suggested reconceptualisation is based on a boundary that surrounds and connects social worker and client, rather than separating the two.

While professional ambitions may attempt to minimise the boundary between client and worker, recent developments point in the opposite direction. 'Responsibilisation' (Rose 2002; Clarke 2005) foregrounds the extent to which micro-systems of accountability are being projected downwards, as being everybody's concern. It is not only professionals but also citizens as service users who are being subjected to new kinds of responsibilisation, delegating more responsibility for planning, service delivery and client outcomes to professionals and service users, while maintaining an overview of activity from a distance through performance indicators and statistical returns (Juhila *et al.* in prep.). What is emphasised here is a combination of an enabling state and active citizens: the state plays a reduced role in the provision of services, and individuals – both professionals and service users – take greater responsibility (Ferguson 2007). Such developments have come with a tighter definition of professional and/or institutional remit but nevertheless a responsibility for anyone involved in the case to draw relevant others' attention to adjacent concerns.

Our interest in boundary work in this chapter is specific in at least two ways. First, while our terrain is that of interactional analysis, much of the work referred to above is based on interviews and focus groups with professionals, concentrating on discussions between professionals, for instance when responding to dilemma scenarios (e.g. Doel *et al.* 2010). Second, our specific interest is in how boundaries are presupposed, touched upon, discussed and negotiated in unfolding contacts with the client or during (interprofessional) group meetings. Meetings between social workers and clients aim to be purposive encounters. The traditional setting for social work encounters, the home visit, is inevitably more informal than the surgery or office. As Margolin (1997: 25) notes, social workers can 'participate in the widest range of conversations, to notice personal relics and bric-a-brac, the most fleeting activities and shifts of mood'. Consumer researchers, too, have suggested that service users did not know exactly what social workers were doing there (Baldock and Prior 1981). Even so, social workers, like other professionals, are expected to have a purpose and focus to their meetings with clients. Kadushin and Kadushin (1997: 140) maintain that the social work interview 'requires some self explication of who we think we are and who we think we represent in this particular situation'. Social workers are inevitably public officials with a remit established by their employment status. This is interactionally evident in, among other features, the allocation of turns in social work meetings: the social worker usually asks the question and the client provides the answer. The social worker can ask about personal details of the client's relationships and expect an answer. The client cannot expect reciprocity. May-Chahal and Har (2011) see social work as inevitably involving 'authorised breaching' of private and interpersonal life, challenging normal conversational conventions of what can be asked. To do so inevitably requires the negotiation of trust (Hall *et al.* 2012) and displays of delicacy (Suoninen, 1999; see also, in this book, Chapter 9 on delicacy), but also establishing the authority to need to know certain things.

Managing purpose and remit comes with the establishing of both focus (centre) and margin (boundary) of attention: what it is that we will concentrate on in particular and what will be considered only more marginally or is left out of the work altogether. In this chapter, we suggest that boundary work is a persistent interactional feature of the social work encounter. Although task or purpose is at times a matter dealt with explicitly at the beginning of the encounter or intervention, our point is more general. Perhaps because of uncertainty of what exactly to expect in the social work encounter, especially when compared to, say, the doctor's visit, which is more tightly structured, we observe a lot of ongoing interaction in which the talkers 'sort out' who does/has done/will do what. Boundary work is about monitoring the flow and scope of activity (and with it, agency). In saying so, we suggest that boundary work is about shaping the social work, delineating the kind of relational work. Both dimensions centrally pertain to the outcomes of social work, the production of enabling identities and social relations. We might suggest that how boundaries are negotiated is a feature of the interaction but is also shaped by context, client category, tasks at hand and so on. For example, it is likely that, while a social worker might try to construct an encounter that is supportive, respectful and purposeful, how this is worked out will vary if the encounter is surrounded by child protection matters or is located in a counselling centre; or if the social worker is intending to take the children into care or supporting a client to manage a personal loss. Issues of coercive/directing and support/enabling frames and footing will be examined throughout the chapter.

Frame and footing

Traditionally, professional practices have been associated with defined roles. 'Role' is indeed the concept that readily comes to mind when talking about a professional mandate that comes with certain expected forms of behaviour and accountability. The underlying assumption is that, through training, contracts and expertise, certain professions take on the responsibility for offering defined services. Along with this go expected forms of role-governed behaviour, scrutiny when people 'step outside' roles, criticism or condemnation when people do not fulfil their role responsibilities, and so on. A simplistic notion of role as mechanistic, anti-individualistic, over-socialised and determined has been the subject of both criticism and debate within social theory (Sarangi and Slembrouck 1996). Some of the key factors in the debate have been that role is flexible, and that it involves role playing – roles are being performed and this involves judgements about what is (in)appropriate behaviour – as well as reflection on the nature of one's conduct. One of the key questions is whether roles are better understood through the interactional constructions through which they come into existence.

As we are interested in how talkers interactionally manage role expectations and constraints, we draw in particular on Erving Goffman's concepts of *frame* and *footing* (Goffman 1974; 1981). A 'frame' is a socially recognised reference for the activity talkers are engaged in: it is both a (shared) definition of a situation and a framework for action (what to do), interpretation (how to interpret actions) and participation (who does what). It comes, among other things, with a set of expectations about likely and allowable interactional behavior and contributions, including the kind of topics talked about and the ways in which the issues raised will be attended to and become consequential. Frames, as Goffman stressed, are both pre-situationally given and situationally established and maintained. The conditions for this reside in interactional behaviour, both verbal (e.g. speaking turns) and physical (e.g. handling of objects, forms of bodily engagement). For example, for a social worker and client to establish the frame of a social work meeting entails that both interlocutors attend to a problem in the client's personal or social situation. They do so by delineating the problem and discussing options, in particular by the social worker asking clarifying questions, establishing expectations and recommending solutions. In contrast, 'footing' has to do with the specific alignment that interactants take up towards the frame, for instance accepting it, displaying reluctance or resisting it (as shown in displays of involvement, commitment or relative distancing). To continue the example above, the social worker is likely to start the conversation and make some reference to what has happened with the problematic situation, in a format that is different from, for example, a meeting with a friend. The clients may align with the social worker's stance and formulation and reach agreements on the way forward. They may resist the formulation, or indeed negotiate the terms under which the topics are talked about. Each of these possibilities is more than the topic being discussed at a particular point in time, as it involves different positioning in the interaction (e.g. a client may resist being drawn into friendly talk and insist on a more formal exchange). To talk about 'changes in footing' invites attention to how interactants in the course of an unfolding encounter manage the fine detail of unfolding role relationships, including their positioning towards one another, and towards the encounter, its categories, goals and objectives.

Footing, therefore, is among other things made manifest at the level of what the talkers say, how they say things and the consequences this has for what happens next in the encounter or for subsequent encounters (in fact, a radical change in footing may transform the nature and scope of the talkers' frame). The scope of a change in footing varies: some changes are short-lived and remain local, as they pertain to subtle shades of tone that apply to a single utterance without lasting implications for a shared definition of the situation. Other changes mark the boundary of an episode. For instance, the shift from troubles-telling to advice-giving (see Chapter 7 on advice-giving) may come with a fundamental distribution in social discursive roles (speaker vs. listener) and thereby constitute a change in frame. So, while Goffman (1981: 128) insisted that 'a change in footing is another way of talking about a change in our frame for events', it is equally instructive to maintain a relative distinction between the two concepts, frame being more oriented to the talkers' definition of the situation and footing bringing out the unfolding dynamics of shifting forms of participation. As Erickson (2004) underlines, participants in interaction bring multiple attributes of their social being to any scene of engagement, and they may make various of these attributes relevant at differing moments during an encounter (e.g. to speak as a spouse, a parent, a client, a tenant).

In conclusion, to say that professionals and clients in interaction display a particular alignment towards a particular definition of the encounter is a discourse analytical way of understanding the situationally amenable aspects of professional and client roles and their boundaries in a particular intervention. It is the alignment the professional seeks to establish with the client that we will draw attention to in our analysis of the data extracts that follow. This alignment is of particular relevance for our understanding of boundary work. Goffman's frame analysis invites attention both to how interactional moves relatively count as actions 'within' a frame (the alignment thus being that the frame is being maintained) and to actions that specifically invite attention to participant attributes or specific understandings of the situation itself. The latter possibility is a key indicator of boundary work taking place.

Boundary work in social work interaction: data examples and analyses

Case 1: 'just points of action that we can both follow and then we know where we are going'

Our first data case underlines these initial observations about boundary work. The excerpt comes from a home visit by a social worker (SW) to a woman (CL) whose mother is suffering from Alzheimer's. The grandmother has recently moved in with her and her two children; she comes from another country, speaks very little English and is isolated as well as confused by her surroundings. The social worker has established a 'community care plan' to support the family and to provide services for the mother. This meeting is the regular review of the plan. There are two excerpts. In the first excerpt immediately below we can note how, at the beginning of the encounter, the focal task at hand is clearly laid out in very formal terms (lines 3–4): the purpose is 'community care assessment'. This particular encounter is one in an 'ongoing process' of review and such is detailed by concentrating on 'objectives', 'how things are going', 'how we go forward' and so on. However, the turn ends with an informal invitation that marks a distinct change in footing: 'So how are you anyway?' (line 8). Attention is moved away from the professional records, as space is first created for the client to voice her experiences since the last visit: things have been going well since, thanks to the social worker's efforts. With this, the client introduces the first actual topic: assistance in finding a home for her mother.

Extract 1

1	SW:	so hello ((client's name))
2	C:	hello
3	SW:	I'm here today just as I explained when I initially came to undertake the community
4		care assessment. I'm here today to do the review as part of ongoing process.
5		the review will just entail sort of looking at some of the objectives that we set out
6		together and just to review them to see how things are going, to see how we go
7		forward or you know to see if we need to change anything or of course to add
8		anything you know to the assessment. So how are you anyway?
9	C:	erm, I'm ok ((laughs)) not bad
10	SW:	good
11	C:	things are going very well, erm, but you've made your best. It is really going very

12		well because, erm, since I talked to you for the first time and you try to find home
13		for my mother, erm, and try to help with the situation to try and rush my mother
14		situation
15	SW:	of course yes

Interaction in the social work encounter is 'set' beforehand by the intervention type, the client and their particular case history. In other data from our corpus of home visits, the professional begins with the statement 'I've got my list of questions' – a list that pertains to this particular client and the worker's professional mission and remit. This suggests an asymmetric relationship, one in which the professional selects the questions asked and the topics talked about, and behind the talk there is a finite list of boxes to be ticked. However, as the extract illustrates, the home visit equally leaves room for negotiation and the introduction of topics and issues by the client, 'So how are you anyway?' cogently epitomising this particular perspective of relative open-endedness. The turn design literally echoes a typical opening move between interactants who are very familiar with one another ('So how have you been?'); it counterbalances the imposing formality of the initial announcement about the institutional task at hand. 'So how are you anyway?' signals that, in addition to the review, there will be room for other things to talk about and issues to attend to. The topic initiative is now with the client. Note how this client responds with a laugh at line 9, suggesting that she notices the possibility for both formal and informal conversation. Such a turn illustrates how the frame definition itself is under scrutiny: the client is reflexively responding and does not allow herself to be 'fooled' by the informality. Interestingly, when she begins to talk she concentrates on formal matters, her mother's care, and not on how she is. This shift in alignment has been short-lived and does not result in a shift in frame.

So far the interaction has concentrated on the positives. This is soon followed by a sequence of troubles-telling, which ends with another change in footing (cf. 'Ok right well' in line 175) as an objective is set and the boundaries of a specific action are being negotiated between the client and the worker. There are two matters to address, neither of which is especially a task for a social worker: applying for a transfer to large accommodation since the mother has arrived and applying for a reduction in the council tax. There is discretion as to what, if any, aspects of these tasks the social worker is to take on. Among other things, the client is to take on the responsibility of completing a form that will reduce the council tax.

Extract 2

160	SW:	well I am really pleased about that so that's one action we've taken that has been
161		quite positive, erm, with regards to the housing that's the next issue, have you
162		heard anything yet?

163	C:	nothing they left me a letter from psychiatrist, erm, I am at the moment this is bad,
164		it's really bad thing because I am expecting a baby in three months. I have 2 kids
165		sleeping in my bed and my mother she is sleeping in a bunk bed she don't have a
166		place to put her clothes and especially because she had problems with getting
167		confused with so she really needs her own room where is her clothes clean clothes and
168		where is the dirty clothes, she must have you know a proper room for her for herself.
169	SW:	yes I understand yes
170	C:	you know so it is really bad. If I had my own money I would rent a house but I'm in
171		a situation I mean financial I am not very good and I don't get any help from my
172		mother at the moment so
173	SW:	ok
174	C:	that is as it is you know
175	SW:	ok right well what I have done I told you I have sent a letter to housing
176	C:	yes yes yes
177	SW:	and supported that and I did mention it to Dr ((name)) as well because Dr ((name))
178		may be able to write a letter of support erm
179	C:	yes
180	SW:	erm, were you going to ask him about that as well because do you remember I
181		mentioned to you about council tax as well?
182	C:	yes
183	SW:	good so yes, so you need to
184	C:	get a form
185	SW:	ok
186	C:	for council tax?
187	SW:	so I'll set that as a new objective you know for next time we meet you know
188	C:	yes yes yes
189	SW:	point of action, just points of action that we can both follow and then we know where
190		we are going
191	C:	yes
192	SW:	so, erm, you submitted the application form anyway to housing?
193	C:	yes
194	SW:	yes so that's done

Particularly in line 175 and following, we can witness the interactional negotiation of a particular division of labour for specific points of action. There are the actions taken by the social worker (line 175: 'sent a letter to housing'; lines 177–178: 'mention it to Dr [name]', who may write a letter of support). These are distinguished from actions to be undertaken by the client (line 180: 'were you going to ask him about that as well' – requesting the letter of support from the psychiatrist; lines 183–186: 'so you need', 'get a form', 'for council tax'; and again in line 192: 'you submitted the application form'). While differentiated between client and worker, these actions are premised on a joint understanding of shared objectives and assessment (see, especially, lines 189–190: 'just points of action that we can both follow and then we know where we are going'). Boundary work here is action oriented – this must be done and who should do it – me, you or someone else. However, the monitoring of roles and responsibilities is not at all fixed beforehand. It is open to negotiation. For instance, a client is likely to be expected to complete a housing application, but in this case the social worker has taken on the role of providing supporting documentation. In the background is an assessment of competencies. In this respect, the social worker is moving between 'offering assistance that can make a difference' (taking care of some of the actions herself) and 'empowering the client' (fostering client capacity). In addition, the task of completing the council tax application is not just a task for the client; it is now an objective on the plan, to be monitored at the next meeting, for which the frame is set and for which the client will be expected to align interactionally in a particular way (e.g. reporting on progress). Typically in social work encounters, there is ongoing attendance to the care plan; its constituent parts can be formally noted across a series of ongoing exchanges. This is one way in which boundaries and associated expectations are displayed, having implications for how the interaction unfolds and how the participants align in the interaction.

Case 2: 'I'm working with you to support you, but I am primarily her social worker'

In our second case the social worker (SW) is visiting a family of a young woman (C) and her child. She has been the subject of serious domestic violence and a child protection plan has been established to protect her and her child from the father. The social services are concerned that the mother does not realise the seriousness of her situation and the dangers to the child; they are considering instituting care proceedings, hence the reference to a legal planning meeting. There are also concerns about the mother's mental health. In the lengthy exchange below, boundary work occurs in the sense that a specific network of support is being interactionally worked up. The social worker begins by drawing a baseline that makes explicit the boundaries of her own work: 'working with you to support you, but I am primarily [the child's] social worker'. The ensuing talk covers a range of allocated workers in detail: an advocate (Maureen), an interpreter (Emma), the domestic violence agency, an under-25 worker (Alison) and a parenting worker (Isobel).

Extract 3

1	SW:	ok ok. But this talk about the legal planning that we were having back in June,
2		basically what it is is you know that I'm Alice's social worker
3	C:	yeah
4	SW:	and I'm working with you to support you, but I am primarily her social worker

5	C:	yeah
6	SW:	what we thought in May would be, it would be a good idea, we thought it would be a
7		good idea if, you remember the ((mental health)) assessments that you went for?
8		remember ((mental health project)) went and once they came here
9	C:	yeah
10	SW:	then you went for your assessment in May. We thought that after this assessment they
11		would say, ok we are going to give her perhaps a ((mental health)) social worker. They
12		didn't do that. So when we went to legal for the meeting in June they said maybe mum
13		should have some support for herself, someone to speak
14	C:	yeah
15	SW:	support mum in meetings, in the conference
16	C:	yeah
17	SW:	you know how you used to bring your mum
18	C:	yeah
19	SW:	that kind of support, but this person would be able to help you understand better what is
20		going on in a way yeah? Even though I explained it to you
21	C:	yeah
22	SW:	this person will be there to support you more than anyone else yeah?
23	C:	yeah
24	SW:	and this person is called an advocate yeah?
25	C:	yeah
26	SW:	that's what they call them, and we found one for you and her name is Maureen and
27	C:	what's she called?
28	SW:	Maureen, Maureen Neil her name is
29	C:	Maureen Neil
30	SW:	Neil. you haven't met her yet, you haven't met her yet
31	C:	oh ok
32	SW:	but we are going to try and arrange for you to meet her in the next couple of weeks
33		before the core group
34	C:	yeah
35	SW:	would that be ok?
36	C:	yeah
37	SW:	but what we are going to do is bring an interpreter just for that meeting yeah?
38	C:	yeah
39	SW:	so that you can understand completely what she is about, what why is she in your life ok?
40	C:	ok
41	SW:	so you've got Emma Carson ok, you've got Emma yeah?
42	C:	yeah
43	SW:	you've got Isobel for parenting. You've got me working with Alice
44	C:	yeah
45	SW:	and working with you but primarily working with Alice. Who else have you got?
46		you've got ((domestic violence agency)). You've got lots actually, you've got quite a
47		big support, I'm trying to think of who else, who else. You've got Alison for the under
48		25s to help you because you were saying you want to go back to school, you want to go

49		back to school. Alison will be the one to help you look at the best way to get back into
50		school. She's got Isobel, who is the parenting worker, remember I just said ok?
51	C:	((inaudible)) she said you were busy and want to meet different people
52	SW:	who said this?
53	C:	Isobel
54	SW:	Isobel yeah, because we've had to put all this support in especially after September,
55		your experiences in September, Alice's experiences in September to make sure nothing
56		happens to harm you or Alice here yeah?
57	C:	yeah
58	SW:	and you've done so well working with services, it's fantastic and you missed ((an
59		appointment with service)) on Saturday didn't you because you weren't well.

The worker's alignment in this exchange is clearly at the meta-level of work. It signals 'I can only do so much', but also 'there is a whole team behind you'. As the child's social worker demarcates her own role (supporting the mother but being primarily the child's social worker), she explains the role of the others in the support network (in one case, there is a specific history of involvement – for example, in lines 10–24, the failed attempt to allocate a mental health social worker to the mother and the client's mother having taken on a support role in representing the client as the context for the current allocation of an advocate). In this way, more than the listing of responsibilities and their boundaries is being accomplished. A participant line of work is laid out by providing a justification for the fragmentation of the work being staged and the client is being prepared for the specific role that the social worker will take on: mostly a coordinator of this network. First of all, there is the more global justification located in the events of September (lines 54–56: 'we've had to put all this support in [. . .] to make sure nothing happens to harm you or Alice here'). In addition, justifications are built around anticipated future events (e.g. line 32: to meet the advocate separately ahead of the core group meeting). From line 45 onwards, the listing of workers involved becomes more exhaustive and there is some light-hearted humour in the listing (line 46: 'You've got lots actually'). The social worker's alignment is reassuring, building client confidence to function within the network (understanding it – who does what, planning around specific actions in the near future, and boosting the client's confidence that she is well taken care of and, more importantly, that she is up to functioning successfully within the network). The client's responses mostly consist of minimal acknowledgement ('yeah'), while querying some detail (e.g. line 51).

However, it is possible to identify the boundary work in the excerpt above as displaying a coercive stance. By emphasising that she is 'primarily' (line 4) the social worker of the child, the social worker is therefore not the social worker of the mother. Perhaps the distinction has been mentioned before (line 15), but now it is being formally established in the identification of an advocate. Although the social worker will explain what is happening at meetings, the advocate is therefore taking on a role that might have been seen as resting with the social worker: 'this person will be there to support you more than anyone else' (line 22). The implication of the description and the title of 'advocate' imply that this person will be on the mother's side, whereas the social worker will not. That the suggestion came from the legal meeting (lines 12–13: 'they said maybe mum should have some support for herself') denoted a new set of formal relations. (This legal meeting refers to the occasion where there is discussion and assessment of the evidence to take the child into care.) The upcoming meeting and possibly the social work–client relationship is changing to a frame involving greater distance, a frame that might turn accusatorial, such as a court with advocates. Note also how the meeting with the advocate is only minimally set up as a choice for the mother: 'would that be ok?' (line 35). Permission is sought in passing and it is not clear whether the mother is invited to agree with the detail of the practical arrangements or the set-up as a whole.

Abbott (1995) called social work a 'profession of boundaries': it attempts to tie together various entities to achieve a defensible jurisdiction, albeit temporary. More than merely working at boundaries, however, social work arguably only comes into existence when the boundaries are being negotiated. In noting this, it is important to examine how the client responds. In this extract, she does not provide an assessment of the attempt at redrawing the boundaries of work; during this exchange the client's contribution is mainly restricted to backchannelling. At lines 27 and 51, the client requests clarification in such a way that it marks an orientation to being attentive to the information provided rather than challenging it or assessing its implications.

Abbott (1995: 558) notes that:

> While the phrase 'boundaries of social work' describes the central determining factors around the profession at any given time, the phrase 'social work of boundaries' captures the idea that local sites of difference always exist from which new professions or sub-professions could emerge.

The point also extends to the work done in interprofessional meetings with its specific challenges of couching the provision of services in collaboration and coordination (Frost *et al.* 2005), as in our third case, immediately below.

Case 3: consensus across boundaries in a core group meeting: 'It's not something that you or grandma are imposing, it's not negotiable'

Interprofessional practice changes the nature of professional talk and interaction. Boundary issues are foregrounded in various ways, as professionals have to engage directly with the diagnostic categories of other professionals, their interventions and the scope of them. As one midwife in our corpus of home visits, 'I'm not an expert but I pick things up.' As they interact in the welfare network, professionals may move the tasks that they take on, necessitating negotiating skills during interprofessional encounters such as the core group meeting. Especially as resources become tighter and services are outsourced, pressure may increase not to take on certain tasks and pass them on to others. Despite responsibilisation (as discussed at the beginning of the chapter), considerable interactional work may thus be invested in moving around interprofessional constraints and opportunities, decision making about where a task is allocated, negotiating what it is and assessing the competencies and capacities involved. The interprofessional context may well encourage the crossing of boundaries and the associated reframing of problems, as is illustrated next.

Our third case has been taken from a core group meeting (such meetings are occasions on which professionals and family members review the child protection plan, monitor progress and decide on required interventions). In the extract below, the social worker (SW), the head teacher (HT) and the school nurse (SN) negotiate on how to address a school-related problem of late arrivals in the morning that is located in the home context: who is to provide help for the mother with the child's behaviour? Is family support work in this area the responsibility of social services or is it something that the school takes a lead in?

Extract 4

1   SW: (. . .) but we need to get this sorted really because I don't know whether, hh, I don't want
2   things to bombard, bombarding C, but what I'm thinking at the moment is that if we had
3   some morning sessions around getting things organised. It's you that needs to be
4   M: yeah. This is it you see. I was saying, you know, she has to be with me full time or it's
5   not going to work
6   SN: are you thinking of observing and see what
7   SW: yeah. Maybe looking at routines and what's going on
8   SN: and giving mum some strategies in a morning
9   mmm. I know, from what, from what I've got from you and I've got an update from
10   ((family support worker)) is that you haven't found that work overly helpful and it's
11   sitting and it's talking and it's, err, and it's not practical
12   SN: no

13	SW:	it's very easy to say what you'd do, but, this is what I'd do because I'm sure you can
14		quite easily give a really good answer how it should be done, but as a reality
15	SN:	yeah ((laughs))
16	SW:	life's not like that and I think that although that work with family support has finished,
17		that we need to look at more really really practical hands on stuff
18	M:	yeah
19	SW:	that C can be involved with and
20	M:	yeah
21	SW:	((headteacher)) was saying that she buys into the, she's buying into the rewards schemes,
22		so I don't want our work to sort of impinge on the parenting course, the referral that's
23		been done, but I think, even something practical around putting the routine, but doing it
24		together with you and C
25	M:	mm, yeah
26	HT:	I said this to grandma that I think that part of the issue with C and I know there's lots of
27		other things going on, is this control. Erm, and sometimes children get to an age where
28		they want to start taking control and if she's got a baby brother, this could be what's
29		happening you know, that she wants to be helping and she wants to be in control of some
30		aspect of her own life
31	M:	yeah
32	HT:	so what I suggested to grandma was that you kind of have that conversation and say,
33		right, you know, you have to be at school by, hh, that's not an option, that's the bottom
34		line, erm so she understands where it's coming from. It's not something that you or
35		grandma are imposing, it's not negotiable

The problem concerns arriving late at school in the mornings. The school nurse challenges the social worker 'are you thinking of observing' (line 6) and 'giving mum some strategies in a morning' (line 8). Whereas the social worker at line 7 initially suggests the possibility of agreement ('Maybe looking at routines and what's going on'), lines 10, 13 and 16 mark her resistance. Three arguments are invoked: this kind of work hasn't been found helpful (line 10), as testified also by the family support worker; it's easy to say what needs to be done, but 'life's not like that' (line 16); and that kind of 'work with family support has finished' (line 16). What is required instead is 'really practical hands on stuff . . . that C can be involved with' (lines 17 and 19). What follows in line 21 redirects interprofessional responsibility: a report from the head teacher that the child is 'buying into the rewards scheme' is proffered by the social worker as an alternative and a practical way forward. Is the problem to remain within the home only? Is there a possibility that it might be co-owned by the school? The pressure is now on the head teacher to respond. Between lines 26 and 35, she responds by recalling an earlier conversation with the grandparent (line 26: 'I said this to grandma'), which suggests the possibility of a co-owned problem context. Two things are noted from that conversation: the remedy is getting the child 'to take control of her own life' (lines 29–30) and a practical way forward can be to instill a school-specific (non-negotiable) value: 'you have to be at school . . . that's not an option, that's the bottom line' (lines 33–34). This way, authority vis-à-vis C is deflected away from the mother and the grandmother, as the school is identified as its sole source: 'It's not something that you or grandma are imposing, it's not negotiable' (lines 34–35). The school-in-the-home is given legitimacy as a source of authority with implications from relations in the home.

Even though interprofessional meetings (e.g. case conferences, core group meetings) can be viewed as constituting an activity-specific frame in their own right (e.g. with expectations of interprofessional consensus being reached as an outcome), they nevertheless come with a multiplicity of complexly layered 'frames of reference' (a category seen from the point of view of 'schooling' is different from one that is seen from the point of view of 'family support'). In the exchange above, the social worker's 'footwork' has succeeded in shifting the problem category from a framework of 'family support' offered by the social services to one of 'schooling'. The talk continues with the mother, father and head teacher agreeing that they will use the reward chart between mum and grandma in order to get C to school. At the end of the exchange (not shown above) the social worker summarises: 'Okay, that's good then, we'll see how that goes yeah (smile). We'll move on to what dad wants to say shortly then, Okay?'. Smiles of agreement were exchanged between all members of the core group indicating consensus that the head's chart proposal would be a good way forward. An entry to this effect was recorded in the social worker's notes. The social worker then moved on to report what the family support worker had suggested – that they reduce their visits. Then she asked dad if there was anything he wanted to say. In doing so, the meeting has implicitly acknowledged the social worker's resistance of any pressure to intervene with perhaps a family support intervention, and it is agreed that, instead, the head teacher and family will work on the reward chart. This way, the head teacher may have taken on a task that could be seen as a social services task (albeit one of family support). In our third case, the professionals' (future) alignment vis-à-vis the diagnostic category and vis-à-vis each other were centrally at stake. As an outcome of the interaction, a future alignment is projected for the parties involved and, more importantly, for C: arriving on time at school in the morning, is 'not something that you or grandma are imposing, it's not negotiable' (lines 34–35).

We don't know from the data available to us the extent to which the actions of the head teacher in stepping beyond her traditional professional boundaries can be seen as an example of 'turf wars' (as discussed at the beginning of the chapter). Will the extra work taken on come with extra resources and will such a responsibility provide a strengthened voice in future discussions of this case or of similar ones? Possibilities are made available by the interprofessional context of the talk. Turf wars are not just waged 'top down'; they are also affected by work that is accomplished 'bottom up'. Boundary work appears to offer opportunities as well as restrictions.

Implications for social work practice

Boundary work is pervasive in social work. It is happening all the time and, when it does, it has consequences both for how the interaction can continue and for establishing the perimeters of the intervention; in short, the nature of what it is the social worker and the client are engaged in and how it evolves interactionally. Boundary work is nearly always both enabling and constraining at the same time. The two dimensions can be identified (with variable emphases) in the three cases we analysed and discussed. In the very first excerpt the constraining effects of the task-oriented opening move by the social worker sets the scene and announces an overall constraint to the encounter; its formal character is subsequently toned down by the plainly conversational 'so how are you anyway', which, although suggesting a freedom for the client to move to any topic of her choice, is responded to (not altogether unexpectedly) with an account of the problem of the grand-mother's care. The detailed boundary work in the second case stresses that the social worker is there for the child (and not the parent). It sets up a potentially conflictive situation that may materialise in subsequent legal meetings (it anticipates formal care proceedings). Roles are thus set up. The social worker's supportive work prepares for the possibility of a legal relationship, which constrains the relationship with the client, though enabling the client through the arrangement of personalised advocacy. In the third case, the interprofessionally negotiated matter of 'who does what' locates a form of family support in an educational rather than a social work intervention. It is enabling by offering a solution, but it also comes with a strong authoritative stance, which is located in the school. Although the exchange's concluding turn is formulated in terms of relieving the (grand)parents of having to invoke their authority ('so she understands where it's coming from. It's not something that you or grandma are imposing'), the imperative that children have to turn up at school on time in the morning arguably extends to the parent (cf. 'it's not negotiable').

It would appear then that social work has a broad palette for developing boundaries in contacts with the client. There is a whole variety of different possibilities in the enabling/constraining continuum, on which social workers can move around quite easily and flexibly. Compared to a doctor or a teacher, the social worker's modes of interaction are much less set. There is a multiplicity of possible frames and corresponding participant alignments that can be put around an encounter and, by implication, around the intervention as it unfolds in time. In each of the three cases, the boundary work has a power dimension in that the social worker attempts to delineate appropriate and timely ways forward. Especially in cases 2 and 3, the change in boundaries is noted as a feature of current circumstances, in both instances implying greater control. The clients' responses are for the most part minimal, with no explicit agreement or disagreement (see Chapter 8 on resistance). This raises the question as to what extent boundary work is the prerogative of the social worker, questioning the success of client empowerment in social work decision making.

In our theoretical introduction we have appealed to the Goffmanian categories of 'frame' and 'footing' as being central to an understanding of boundary work. What exactly, then, is the relationship between the three concepts? It is worth noting here that frame is, of course, a spatial metaphor. As an enacted definition of the situation and its participant relationships, it frames (puts a frame around) the encounter and with it the intervention. By applying the term simultaneously in the sense of a 'frame of reference' and a 'frame within which to act', the concept of frame suggests that there is an intimate relationship between professional knowledge and understanding and ways of interacting. The two cannot really be separated from one another. Professional understandings of a situation come with interactional constraints, while interactional developments shape professionally relevant understandings. In short, we have been using frame and footing as analytic concepts because we want to underline the interactional constitution of professional boundary work. Our justification for the title of this chapter, 'boundary work' (rather than frame analysis), has been that the concept is used in the professional literature and is often seen in a wide range of procedures, guidance, policies and paperwork. In contrast we have shown that boundaries are much wider than the professional literature suggests as they are an ongoing and pervasive feature of everyday social work encounters and formulations. The problem of boundaries cannot be solved by producing yet another guidance note. As Ayre (2001: 893) notes:

> It is not just the depth of the pile of guidance notes which causes concern, it is also their texture, in that they have become ever more closely woven. If an instance of error seems to have fallen through the net provided by existing guidance, we start to write on the spaces between the lines in the vain hope that we will eventually catch everything.

6

NARRATIVE

Christopher Hall and Maureen Matarese

Narrative and storytelling are widely recognised as central to social interaction. People tell stories to explain, entertain and convince others in a wide variety of contexts. Unsurprisingly narrative is also central to social work and in recent years has been the subject of a number of developments in social work theory and research. Talk between social workers and clients is analysed as narrative (Marvasti 2002; Hyden and Overlien 2005; Hall *et al.* 2006). Research on talk between professionals draws on narrative approaches (Crepeau 2000; White 2002; Riemann 2005), as does writing in social work files (Hall 1997; Hall *et al.* 2006; White *et al.* 2009). Interview data between researchers and service users and social workers is seen as narrative (Hall 1997; Martin 1998; Wells 2010). Furthermore, narrative is increasingly featured in social work education (Rutten *et al.* 2010), with social workers encouraged to think of their practice in narrative ways (Baldwin 2013). Particular social work methods draw on narrative (White and Epston 1990; Parton and O'Byrne 2000; Roscoe *et al.* 2011). This chapter will examine what developments in the study of narrative and storytelling can offer to the study and practice of social work. In particular we concentrate on approaches that examine narratives told in everyday social work encounters. For example:

```
1  C:    (.) she surprises me because one day I was asleep on the sofa and I wake her
2        and then she said goodbye I'll have a bath and I was like in shock because
3  SW:   oh good good
4  C:    so slowly she is coming, you know, small things she is coming, something
5        I never let my mother have a bath because she doesn't know whether it is
6        hot or cold
7  SW:   I see
8  C:    it's a safety thing you know she doesn't feel pain
```

Above a daughter (C) describes to the social worker (SW) recent improvements in her mother's condition now she has better medication. In this extract, the daughter illustrates this with a narrative of an incident of her mother taking a bath by herself. The story is told from the daughter's perspective; she was asleep and her mother told her she was going for a bath (lines 1 and 2). However, the daughter considered that perhaps the social worker had not understood the significance of the story, so explains why it was important: until now she would not let her take a bath without supervision (lines 5 to 8).

Definitions of narrative and story

A narrative is when a narrator tells a listener a connected series of events to communicate an experience or point of view. As Riessman and Quinney (2005: 394) put it: 'sequence and consequence: events are selected, organized, connected and evaluated as meaningful for a particular audience'. Although different approaches emphasise different aspects of narrative, there are some commonalities. Narrative suggests a temporal aspect to talking, writing and thinking, usually with a beginning, middle and end. The events in question are organised in such a way that the resulting narrative has consequences for both the narrator and listener/reader. It implies a move from one state of affairs to another, and in doing so makes a point.

Some writers make conceptual distinctions between narrative and story, especially in literary theory, and the etymology of the words is interesting. Narrative is associated with an authoritative telling of events, whereas storytelling is associated with entertaining an audience, setting up an interesting challenge for the audience as to the truthfulness of the story. In the social sciences the use of the terms is less precise, so in this chapter they are used interchangeably.

Narrative in the social sciences

While narrative theory and analysis have traditionally been associated with literary studies, over the last 30 years theory, research and practice drawing on narrative have flourished across the social sciences. Narrative approaches to data collection and analysis are now a constituent part of (mainly) qualitative research methods, some directly applying concepts from literary theory to talk and interaction in a wide variety of contexts. However the 'narrative turn' in the social sciences has been so far reaching that writers discuss narrative from widely different and sometimes contradictory positions. For some, narratives are identified in everyday talk and interaction. Others see narrative as located in the psychology of the individual – 'the storied self' (McAdams 1996). For some, narrative is a feature of wider cultural formations. For others the focus of the analysis is the text itself.

While offering a wide range of possibilities for the researcher, it is often hard to compare writers' different theoretical foundations. Furthermore, the popularity of narrative has resulted in publications in which any form of talk that recounts past events, especially interview data, is referred to as narrative, even when no narrative analysis is attempted (Atkinson 1997; Riessman 2008).

This chapter concentrates on narrative as a way of understanding social work. We describe some of the key theoretical concepts developed in the social sciences; in particular, we compare approaches that examine narrative in terms of identity, structure and performance. We then provide examples of how narratives in social work interaction can be analysed.

The key concepts in narrative theory are *identity*, *temporal structure* and *performance*. Ezzy (1998: 246) links the three concepts together in the work of Ricoeur: 'Narrative identity is coherent but fluid and changeable, historically grounded but "fictively" reinterpreted, constructed by an individual but constructed in interaction and dialogue with other people.'

These three concepts explore different aspects of narrative: is the orientation of the research to the narrator, the text or the storytelling occasion?

Narrative identity

It is suggested that the stories we tell enable us to display and establish our narrative identity. Ricoeur (1991: 29) sees narrative as enabling us to gain a sense of ourselves, 'life as an activity and passion in search of a narrative'. By creating and performing stories we are able to establish a coherent sense of who we are and at least, for the time being, we can create self-understanding. Indeed, we understand the world and ourselves through stories; life and narration depend on one another: 'Subjects recognise themselves in the stories they tell about themselves' (Ricoeur 1988: 247). Narrative enables us to understand the world around and also offers ways to act in and on the world:

> Our life, when then embraced in a single glance, appears to us as the field of a constructive activity, borrowed from narrative understanding, by which we attempt to discover and not simply to impose from outside the *narrative identity which constitutes us*.
>
> (Ricoeur 1991: 32)

Such an orientation has been developed by Bruner (2004: 692): 'we seem to have no other way of describing "lived time" save in the form of narrative'. Bruner's work has been particularly important in narrative psychology and life story methods, perhaps the most widespread development of narrative in the social sciences. It also links to the temporal aspect of narrative, as people develop continuity in their lives by adding new narratives, which they use to organise the past and are available to understand the future (van Nijnatten 2010: 10).

While narrative psychology espouses a constructed nature of narrative, the analysis aims to say something about the storyteller, rather than the storytelling occasion. Edwards (1997: 272) notes that '[narrative psychology] takes one step back from events themselves and takes a psychological interest in the speaker. It treats people's discourse as how they 'see' things ... whether as representatives of groups or cultures, or as individuals.'

Discourse analytic approaches also locate identity within talk and interaction; however, they do not attempt to 'read through [stories] to the life beyond' (Edwards 1997: 271). Instead, identity is seen as constructed in the talk. De Fina and Schiffrin (2006: 2) describe four features of identity as a process:

> (1) it takes place in concrete and specific interactional occasions, (2) yields constellations of identities instead of individual, monolithic constructs, (3) does not simply emanate from the individual, but results from processes of negotiation and entextualization that are eminently social and (4) entails 'discursive work'.

Antaki and Widdicombe (1998: 3) provide a similar list of identities being constructed and made consequential in interaction, but also note that identities in talk rely on the negotiation of categories and the associated attributes (see Chapter 3 on categorisation).

These approaches to identity in narrative are clearly different from social work formulations, traditionally associated with ego psychology; as Miehls and Moffatt (2000: 342) note, identity 'is constructed in terms of inter-subjectivities rather than through intrapsychic processes'. This is not to suggest there is no room for a psychology of the self (Wetherell 2007), but this focus on the ways identities are constructed enables concentration on the active ways in which both social worker and clients are involved in producing versions of themselves as a central part of their interaction.

There are a number of criticisms of narrative psychology and life story approaches that rely on interview methods to elicit data to investigate narrative identity. Stokoe and Edwards (2006: 57) are particularly critical of the biographical approach, which they describe as 'a contrived situation based on the assumption that their "life stories" and experiences are readily available to "dump" from memory'. Atkinson (1997: 327) sees narrative research as a 'mixed blessing . . . often sentimental and romantic', and warns against privileging the narrative as a special kind of representation. Woods (2011: 401) questions the instruction of the narrative researcher: 'Tell us your story, because it is true (to the human condition), because it is yours (an authentic expression of your individual experience), and because it is good for you (as part of the healing process).' In the light of such criticisms, the more modest claims of discourse approaches to narrative in talk and interaction have much to offer.

Narrative structure

The way narrative is temporally structured is the subject of important writing. Ricoeur sees narrative as offering ways in which people make sense of events around them and turn those reflections into action: he asks 'in what way is the ordinary experience of time, borne by daily acting and suffering, refashioned by its passage through the grid of narrative' (1985: 249). The temporal characteristic of narrative enables storytellers to give significance to past events in the present situation and has the potential to endure in future narrative performances. The key concept is 'emplotment': events that might appear unconnected are taken from the teller's experience and synthesised into a unified and complete story. It is 'drawing configuration out of a succession' (Ricoeur 1991: 22).

Narrative structure involves an orientation to the form rather than the content of the story. The influence of literary theory is evident with attempts to develop concepts such as plot, character, genre and point of view in the analysis of talk and interaction. However, the key feature is how narrative is structured in such a way that it is consequential for the audience. The narrator needs to consider what aspects of the situation are included in the narrative and what are left out, and how the events fit into a plot that the listener/reader can recognise.

These approaches tend to concentrate on the narrative as a text, an artefact to be analysed in itself rather than concentrating on the narrator or storytelling occasion. However, the narrative is not just a list of events but is organised in such a way as to address an audience. Sometimes the audience is specifically addressed and is clearly identifiable; other times it is a general audience. In order to keep the audience involved, the narrative needs to address a number of tasks, for example to make a point, to be intelligible, not to be repetitive, and to have a sense of drama.

The most celebrated model for examining narrative structure is provided by the sociolinguist, William Labov (1972). He was interested in how the stories of African American adolescents could be seen as having a coherent structure. He provides an ideal structure of a 'fully formed narrative', based on the temporary organisation of the clauses in the speech. There are six elements: an *abstract*, which introduces the gist of the story to come; an *orientation*, which sets the scene; a *complication*, which introduces the problem or rupture in routine affairs; an *evaluation*, which indicates the significance of the event; a *resolution*, which deals with the problem; and a *coda*, which rounds off the story. A verbal sequence of clauses in the story is matched to a sequence of events organised temporally. Such a structure provides both causality and credibility to the story, and is organised to counter what Labov calls the 'so what' question. The evaluation in particular is a direct address to the audience that events happened in the way they did and were (and are) important.

Riessman (2008) uses the Labovian model to understand how divorced people talk about relationship breakdown and make sense of their marital problems. She considers that the organisation of events in the stories and the significance given to them uncovers displays of distress that would not have been possible through an analysis of the themes in the talk. McDaniels (1995) examines how adults struggled to make sense of chaotic circumstances during their childhood by examining the use of various forms of evaluation in narratives to display the significance of events. Usita *et al.* (1998) uses narrative coherence to examine how people with Alzheimer's disease struggle to organise the chronology of their stories.

In contrast to Labov's narrow view of what constitutes a narrative, Gee (1991) provides a broader approach to examining narrative structure. He is concerned with identifying how parts or topics of long stretches of life story interviews fit together, using the poetic feature of tone and voice, and displaying shifting temporal structures. His analysis identifies the narrative coherence in a life story told by a woman suffering from schizophrenia, in what at first appears to be incoherent talk. Poindexter (2002) shows how different methods of addressing the structure of interview data uncovered different meanings. For example, by adding to Gee's model a concern with the co-construction aspects of the storytelling (for example, incomplete turns), more complex explanations emerge of the structure of the story, including affiliation between narrator and listener. Applying concepts of narrative structure provides important insights into how people describe and manage stressful situations by revealing the complexity of meanings on which narrators draw.

Narrative performance

The third concept associated with narrative is performance, the story as told to an audience, and constructed in terms of 'ratified hearers' (Goffman 1981). In contrast to studies of narrative structure, research on narrative performance concentrates on the telling of the story rather than the story itself. There is a tradition in literary theory of locating the understanding of the text in the interpretation of the reader (Iser 1974) or, as Fish (1980) calls it, the 'interpretative community'. In the social sciences, the work of discourse analysts sees the story as constructed in the interaction between the teller and listener, produced for and with the present listener to manage the dilemmas of a particular encounter. As Goodwin and Heritage (1990: 299) say: 'Rather than treating stories as self-contained cultural artefacts, conversation analysts have stressed the way stories are structured with respect to the contingencies of the interaction in which they are embedded.'

Sacks (1992) analysed stories in conversation as one form of talk-in-interaction. A central feature of everyday conversation, as described in Chapter 2, is its organisation in terms of sequences of talk, for example questions and answers, invitation and acceptance/rejection and so on. To make space to tell a story, the storyteller needs to create an agreement to talk for an extended period without an interruption. This requires a 'story preface', an announcement of an intention or request to tell a story, for example 'I must tell you what happened to me the other day.' The listener is therefore constrained from interrupting until the story is completed, for example with a closing comment such as 'so that's what happened'. The aim is therefore to study 'how stories are told and what conversational actions are accomplished in their telling' (Stokoe and Edwards 2006). It is not a concern to identify what is or is not a narrative; instead, it is an interest in how the participants treat the interaction as a storytelling occasion, by the nature of the turn allocation and the negotiation about its significance (Edwards 1997: 273).

The story recipient is therefore important in the analysis of the story. As Gubrium and Holstein (1998: 178) say, 'listeners are often active co-participants in both the elicitation and production of stories, working with the machinery of ordinary conversation to shape storytelling'. This is in contrast to approaches that do not include the consideration of the listener in their analysis, particularly the activities of the interviewer. The story recipient is important in a number of ways. First, stories are told to particular audiences and inevitably the narrator will organise the story in terms of anticipating the listener's reaction. Second, listeners can provide 'continuers' (mm hm, uh huh, yeah) to encourage the teller to keep talking and, if they do not, may disrupt the storytelling. The storyteller may make direct appeals to shared understanding of the salience of the story: 'you know what I mean'. Third, the storyteller is likely to indicate their orientation to the events of the story. They may also display their legitimacy to tell the story, the trusted teller of the tale (Shuman 2006), by, for example, indicating their presence at the incident or expertise on the topic. Smith (1993) indicates how a student describes her friend's mental illness and provides preliminary instructions as to how the story should be heard. For example, she states 'I was the last to admit that she was becoming mentally ill', thereby indicating that the fact of the mental illness was independent of her recognition, therefore she was not complicit in its identification. Apart from addressing the potential 'so what' question, the storyteller faces a wide range of interactional challenges in terms of accountability and credibility.

Fourth, at the end of the story the listener reacts to the appropriateness or significance of the story. If this does not occur there are likely to be interactional consequences. Stivers (2008: 34–35) makes a distinction between alignment, referring to the listener's stance to the activity in progress, and affiliation, 'meaning that the hearer displays support of and endorses the teller's conveyed stance'. Responses such as 'that's fantastic' or 'I see' are assessments of the story. Sacks *et al.* (1974) considers that the story preface informs the listeners of the preferred response to the story.

The evaluation clause in the Labov model implies an attention to the reaction of a listener, actual or idealised. However, there are criticisms of Labov's analytic scheme: that it is concerned with what a story 'ought to contain', in advance of examining specific instances; and that the categories 'impose rather than reveal' features of narrative (Edwards 1997: 276). It is the case that everyday interaction is likely to involve more complex methods of story preface and the negotiation of speaking turns. Conversational stories, in particular, are rarely personal in the sense of belonging to a single speaker or bounded by formal structures. Instead, they are co-constructed, contested and constituted in relationships, often characterised by challenges, questions, clarifications and speculations (Crepeau 2000; Ochs and Capps 2001). One story is often responded to with another story (Sacks 1992) as the second narrator demonstrates his/her understanding of the significance of the first story.

Narratives told in institutional settings are likely to have a more discrete structure. The allocation of roles of narrator and listener are likely to be established with particular kinds of stories following partially predetermined storylines. In court, narratives are restricted in the sense that the storyteller is encouraged to tell the temporary flow of the events but is prevented from indicating their significance. Gubrium and Holstein (1998) examine questioning by a district attorney of a potential involuntary psychiatric patient. The district attorney starts a question-and-answer sequence, but then refuses to take the next allotting turn, thereby forcing the potential patient to extend and elaborate her story. As Gubrium and Holstein (1998: 177) summarise, 'narrative production is necessarily collaborative, even while it is institutionally informed'.

In the illustrations that follow involving social work settings, we will consider in particular how storytelling turns are allocated. We will examine how features of institutional or conversational storytelling are recognisable: is the storyteller interrupted; is the story co-constructed or responded to with second stories? In particular we are interested in how the listener, usually the social worker, assesses the client's story and the consequences for the ongoing interaction.

Narrative and storytelling in social work interaction: data examples and analyses

An invited story

Invited stories are typical of social work interactions, as the social worker invites the client to report on a particular set of circumstances. This is often formulated in terms of what has happened to the client since the last meeting with the social worker. Invited stories have been examined by Watson (1990: 276), who notes that 'the teller of an invited story has to tell the story the recipient wants, and has asked to hear'. The social worker and client are likely to anticipate a report on social work-related matters, even when the invitation is open-ended. For example, in an opening to a home visit to a woman whose mother has dementia (examined in detail in Chapter 5, Extract 1), the social worker provides a formal introduction to identify the purpose of the meeting, but then provides an open story invitation 'so how are you anyway?' It signals openness and informality but is still responded to by the client in terms of the task at hand, the care of her mother.

In Extract 1 below, the social worker provides a specific topic for the invited story. The case involves a mother (M) and her two daughters. The mother has been suffering from mental health problems and has had difficulty taking the children to school on time. The social worker (SW) is in a child welfare team in the UK and had been working with the family for about a year.

Extract 1

1	SW:	so first day back at school, how did it go?
2	M:	good
3	SW:	yeah
4	M:	got there (2) well we were strolling but when we got there we saw someone and she was
5		like cos like 'have they've gone in' and she goes 'yeah' and we started running, we got
6		there but ((child's)), well everyone was everywhere so it didn't really matter she weren't
7		late still ten to nine and they were just [starting] to go in and ehm she seemed
8	SW:	[°good°]
9	M:	alright going in, that was it, waved her off, 'see you ((child)) love you bye' picked her
10		up from school (2) and I didn't know which teacher or you know I was just waiting
11		but ehm I didn't meet the teacher I met the teacher's assistance assistant and asked,
12		I said I've come to get ((child)) and went 'that's all right I'll tell the teacher'
13		so that was that, ((child)) said it was alright
14	SW:	[°yeah°]
15		(3)
16	M:	see yeah
17	SW:	yeah cos I mean six weeks is quite a long time isn't it getting out of the routine that
18		you'd had worked quite hard to get in to, so how was getting up this morning?

This story invitation is the first exchange in the interview. Given the background to the case, the social worker might be anticipating that the start of a new school year puts pressure on the mother. The story invitation in line 1 is therefore specific but also draws on a mutual understanding of a familiar set of circumstances: 'the first day back', formulated as a potential problem. The mother responds in line 2: 'good'. However, the story invitation is unfulfilled. The response 'yeah' (line 3) reiterates the invitation. At line 4 the mother begins the story: 'Got there'. This is followed by a two-second pause, which in other interactions would have signalled a transfer of speaker slot, but here the storyteller is able to keep the floor. We can see, therefore, that the story invitation and preface has been negotiated, with the listener (the social worker) instrumental in establishing expectations.

The story from line 4 to line 13 is accomplished with only two quiet continuers by the social worker (line 8 and 14), which do not produce any pause in the storytelling. The structure displays elements of a Labovian model. There is an abstract 'Got there' (line 4); an orientation 'we were strolling' (line 4); a complication 'they've gone in' (line 5); a resolution 'she weren't late' (lines 6–7); and an evaluation 'she seemed alright going in' (lines 7 and 9). There is a drama in the story with anxiety when they found out that they might be late. The tension is illustrated with reported speech between the mother and perhaps another parent (see Chapter 10 on reported speech). There is an interesting ending to the story. The evaluation, 'she seemed alright' focuses the success of the story on the child's response to the drama, which is illustrated with more reported speech, 'wave her off "see you [child] love you bye"' (line 9). It appears to be a normal farewell at the school gate. However, we hear nothing of the anxiety that the rush had created for the mother, and the completion is justified in terms of the child's feelings. Furthermore, the story is told in terms of 'we' rather than 'I'. This raises an interesting question over the status of clienthood, since much of the focus of the social worker's work has been the mother's coping with everyday child care demands.

The other interesting feature is that, without an assessment by the social worker, the mother tells a second story about the end of the school day. It reports a meeting with the teaching assistant that also appeared to go well (lines 10–13). Note how the second story follows immediately on from the first without additional invitation from the social worker or hesitation from the mother.

At the end of the second story, there is a three-second pause, but the social worker does not take this next turn. The mother produces a possible ending to the story 'see yeah' (line 16) and the social worker now assesses the story (lines 17–18). However, the assessment does not comment on the story itself that has just been told but its overall significance in the mother's strategies for getting the child to school on time. In this sense it is a meta-comment, 'have you re-established appropriate coping strategies', rather than an affiliation with the drama of the story. The social worker now invites another story about getting up.

A story as an illustration

Extract 2 is from a home visit by a social worker in a child welfare team in the UK (SW) to the grandmother of a child who has special educational needs (GM). The grandmother is looking after her grandson and wishes to take on the status of his guardian. This involves a court application and the social worker is visiting to complete the appropriate forms. Inevitably the home visit involves many questions about the family history and the child's development. While there is considerable talk about the past, this is often in the form of general information and recollection, for example 'was he a healthy baby? Yes, he was a gorgeous baby.' Sometimes such questions are answered with a story.

In the extract below, the social worker is talking about the child's recent progress at school and the plan to identify his educational needs through a 'statement' (a formal assessment to identify educational needs and appropriate resources).

Extract 2

1	SW:	and kind of, I'm so pleased that they were saying he's (1) ehm he's now taking part in
2		group sessions [group] work
3	GM:	[yes] yeah
4	SW:	and he's talking, he's obviously talking about himself which I think I wouldn't have
5		expected him to do that
6	GM:	no
7	SW:	no
8	GM:	[no]
9	SW:	[because] when he did I was shocked
10	GM:	yeah and I was delighted the other day when I went to pick him up from school we had a
11		misunderstanding it had stopped raining and so he decided he was walking home (.) and
12		so I picked him up halfway and he was walking with two pals and I was really really
13		thrilled that he was walking with two pals (.) you know and it's one of them is a chap that
14		he goes to youth club with and the other one is somebody he knew at ((school)) and you
15		know I was really pleased to see that because he's usually just on his own
16	SW:	and when I spoke to ((mother)) yesterday she was saying that she she can see that
17		he is happy and that he is settled and she doesn't want to disrupt that so
18	GM:	yeah
19	SW:	that's really positive that she can ehm see that and obviously all this stuff, having this
20		stability now for him and having ((therapist)) going in and supporting his emotional
21		development we can really kind of hopefully things are moving forward for him and
22		getting a statement

The social worker relates comments from a recent meeting with the school at which they describe how the child was taking part in group sessions and hence he was talking about himself (lines 1–5). This is depicted as an unexpected but a positive development. Although the social worker describes a past event, a meeting at the school, the comment only hints at a story, since there are no specific events described nor is there a movement from one state of affairs to another. The key feature of this talk is proposing a potential assessment of the child's progress; it is a meta-formulation.

In contrast, the grandmother tells a detailed narrative about the child walking home from school with friends (lines 10–15). It is personal, being told from her own observations and reporting personal reactions: I saw this, I was really pleased. Again there are elements of a Labovian structure: an abstract: 'delighted . . . when I went to pick him up from school' (line 10); an orientation: 'misunderstanding, it had stopped raining' (line 11); and a complication: 'he was walking with two pals' (line 12). The evaluation and resolution are, however, confusing. The key contrast in the story is that normally he walks from school alone but on this occasion he was with friends. However, the first part of the contrast is not specified until the end (line 15). Perhaps the lack of acknowledgement from the social worker, for example at the pause on line 11 or 'you know' at line 13, forces the grandmother to emphasise the contrast that had only been implied until then.

In contrast to Extract 1, there is more of an assessment of the narrative by the social worker (lines 16–22), as he tells a second story. Sacks (1992) considers that in everyday interaction second stories are an efficient way of displaying affiliation; however, in professional–client interaction, a second story is less likely to be based on personal experiences. Ruusuvuori (2005: 205) found only one example in a corpus of 228 troubles-telling sequences that she sees as abandoning the professional role. Professionals affiliated with the patients' circumstances at a general level without equivalent personal experiences. Here, however, the social worker's second story reports a conversation with the child's mother in which she also sees that the child is happy and settled (line 17). It does not include personal reactions of the social worker like that of the grandmother, but is used to add to the number of people who are noticing the child's improvement. It only hints at a contrast between the mother's current view of the child being happy now and perhaps a less favourable view of the child's situation at a previous time. The assessment of these stories, as with Extract 1, is aimed at the overall state of affairs of the child, rather than the drama of either of the stories told.

An accountable story

The following two extracts come from scheduled post-case conference meetings between two separate homeless clients with their shelter caseworkers in the US. As such, these extracts differ greatly from earlier ones in several marked ways. First, the former extracts come from home visits, while the latter were taken from an urban homeless shelter context, in which meetings were held on-site. The former extracts provide examples of calm interaction, and what is relevant about these narratives is different: these former narratives are important in part because of the evaluation the social worker provides of the client's narrative. The social worker actively engages in assessing these narratives, whereas, in the latter extracts, the caseworkers' engagement in the clients' narratives is quite different, and the talk is rather agitated.

In Extract 3, a client (C) is upset because someone at the shelter has stolen his phone, and though the narrative is irrelevant to the client's case, the caseworker (CM) allows him to provide a narrative, in part to provide a rationale for his assessment of himself as a target of injustice at the shelter.

Extract 3

1	CM:	Henry, it's just our regular <u>meet</u>ing.
2	C:	yeah, I got my phone stolen again.
3	CM:	Henry, every w[eek you
4	C:	[A. S. P. ((organisation he is blaming for stealing the phone))
5	CM:	every wee[k,
6	C:	[A.
7	CM:	listen to (.) me (.).
8	C:	okay.
9	CM:	before you say anything.
10	C:	okay.
11	CM:	<every week, you're getting your phone stole>.=
12	C:	=no.
13	CM:	>I don't understand.<
14	C:	I am a target. (.) I am a target to the ((shelter)), and I am a target to staff, I am a target
15		now listen to <u>this</u>, I'm going to the <u>bus</u> stop the other day,
16	CM:	okay.
17	C:	that's two days ago (.) Alright. the bus comes an I'm annoyed with the bus driver
18		cause he wouldn't let me off one day he wouldn't let me <u>off</u> where I wanted to get
19		<u>off</u>. Anyway, the puddle was out there, (.) I was up on the sidewalk when the bus
20		almost hits me and drenches me. I went nuts. Alright? Well, <u>he</u> wouldn't open the
21		door to the bus, so I went into the building, right?
22	CM:	okay?
23	C:	called police. Okay? ((Shelter)) let me in. There was a girl and the guy. Who's the
24		62-year-old worker over there?
25	CM:	the six[ty
26	C:	[he's 62 years old, (.) mustache, slim,
27	CM:	[XXXX ((indistinguishable))
28	C:	[He works here, yes. He works here.
29	CM:	what <u>time</u> was it?

30	C:	it was night time. No it was <u>morning</u>.
31	CM:	he's a <u>work</u>[er?
32	C:	[yup ehh 9 o'clock in the morning. Well, he said, 'What's Henry doin
33		in here? Get him the hell outta here! Who let Henry in here? blah blah blah' I'm
34		looking at this guy—what is his <u>problem</u>! Right? Anyway he turns to me and he
35		goes "SO what! You <u>deserved</u> it!" De<u>serv</u>ed it? Anyway XXXX but I got
36		something for him. I'd like to know <u>why</u> he did that, I was hoping to see him to<u>day</u>.

The first observation one might make is that Henry works diligently to initiate his narrative in lines 2, 4 and 6. In line 11, the caseworker suggests that Henry, the client, often has his phone stolen, and Henry provides a dispreferred response that does not affiliate or develop rapport with her. His bald on-record 'No' initiates a comment from the caseworker 'I don't understand.' This acts as a clarification request, which Henry orients to by providing a narrative that accounts for his statement. Accounts often manage the space between expectation and action (see Chapter 4 on accountability), and in this case his account justifies her expectation that his phone is always getting stolen with the reality: his phone is stolen often because he feels that he is a target at the shelter. In line 14, he provides an orientation for his narrative, locating his story in the context of him being a target at the shelter. He uses a pre-sequence 'listen to this' (line 15) to prepare his caseworker for his story, and then orients her through timing language ('two days ago'). He provides a narrative that functions to describe the injustice done to him, using words such as 'Alright?' and 'Right?' to seek affiliation from his caseworker. The caseworker does seem to follow his lead, using discourse markers such as 'okay' to allow Henry to continue using the floor. She also asks follow-up questions that function to allow Henry to elaborate his story in lines 32–36.

Like the previous extracts, this narrative includes parts of the Labovian narrative structure, including: an abstract: 'Listen to this'; orientations: 'I am a target' and 'two days ago'; a complicating action when the puddle drenches him; a secondary complicating action (getting yelled at by the worker); an evaluation: 'I got something for him'; and a potential conclusion: 'I was hoping to see him today'. Interestingly, the caseworker's back-channelling (e.g. 'okay') facilitates the completion of this narrative whole, which tells us that the caseworker was invested in allowing him to tell the whole story. However, as the first portion of the narrative (regarding the puddle) is never concluded and as the second portion of the narrative (regarding the shelter worker) is on a different subject, it is also possible that these are two separate narratives that both work to establish Henry's position as 'a target'. He was a physical target when he was splashed by the water, and he was a target of the worker's anger. If this is the case, then both narratives include some traditional elements of narrative structure, though not all, and they together function to categorise him as 'a target'. Although he never returns to the issue of his stolen phone, these categorising narratives serve to provide evidence for the credibility of his argument that his phone is also stolen because he is a target, as he was in these other incidences. When the narrative ended, the caseworker allows him to tell several other short narratives before using 'okay' to shift to a new topic. She does not engage with the story but continues on to discuss his case as a whole, again emphasising her attention to his *need* for storytelling without actually engaging in the stories themselves.

An institutional story

The final extract reveals a slightly different type of narrative. While the previous extracts highlighted personal narratives in social work meetings, this extract presents a client who tries to claim specific knowledge (called 'epistemic authority' by Heritage and Raymond 2005) about the shelter by claiming access to an institutional narrative. He, however, does so unsuccessfully, and the shelter caseworker reclaims authority over this narrative through her own telling of the story. While a personal narrative tells a story specific to an individual (as seen in previous extracts), an institutional narrative, in this case, presents stories that index tropes common to the shelter experience. In this case, the institutional narrative the client engages in relates to a shelter policy emphasising increased responsibility. The policy required shelter caseworkers to expedite homeless clients' movement through the shelter system by holding them more accountable for their responsibilities. Juhila *et al.* (in prep.) refer to this as *responsibilisation*: a situation in which policy-level demands for increased responsibility trickle down to impact on responsibilities emphasised in everyday practice. This client, who had exceeded the maximum time limit for shelter stay, was trying to prove knowledge of this trope by telling the narrative of that institutional process.

Extract 4

1	C:	cause the pressure's on <u>her</u>, right?
2	CM:	right, the pressure'[s on basically all of us.
3	C:	[technically technically. (.) Okay, technically, technically when
4		you <u>come</u> in the door that's what what's that? (.) the IPO or whatever,=
5	CM:	=I-L-P
6	C:	I-L-P. (.) That's suppose to take your place, so by the time you're nine months due
7		you're supposed to be, (.)
8	CM:	but it's not supposed to [be
9	C:	[I know.=

10	CM:	=Lemmie lemmie explain something to you. (.) It's only supposed to be three
11		months,
12	C:	right
13	CM:	that you're supposed to be in the shelter.
14	C:	exactly
15	CM:	you been here <u>nine</u>.
16	C:	right
17	CM:	okay. Um so the pressure IS on now because this is <u>not</u>, what <u>happened</u> is (.) it
18		took (.) <people started to make this into a <u>home</u>.>
19	C:	exactly
20	CM:	they started living here <u>26</u> years, <u>10</u> years, <u>5</u> years, <u>4</u> years, and <it was never
21		supposed to happen.> Things fell through the tracks.
22	C:	XXXX ((indistinguishable))
23	CM:	right. Things fell through the <u>cracks</u>. (.) Fine. So now the pressure's on <u>us</u>. Yes,
24		the Mayor <u>do</u> have a five (.) year plan to bring down homelessness and <u>yes</u> he's on
25		our case just cause he wants to look <u>good</u>. So heads will <u>roll</u>.
26	C:	mm-hmm
27	CM:	so we have to put the pressure on <u>you</u> guys unfortunately you've been here for
28		nine months, (.) so now the pressure's on. it's not like you've been here for <u>si:x</u>,
29	C:	no, I can handle [the pressure
30	CM:	[right.

This extract begins with the client claiming epistemic access to the ins and outs of the shelter by claiming to know who, specifically, receives pressure from the administration. His claim, however, is threatened by his use of the tag question 'right', which while aligning with his caseworker also downgrades his epistemic authority, establishing her as having more epistemic authority than him (Heritage and Raymond 2005). While the caseworker uses 'right' (line 2), seemingly acknowledging and validating his claim, she then alters the characterisation of the pressure significantly.

In line 3, the client interrupts his caseworker, trying to initiate his telling of the institutional narrative that explains the process clients should follow. However, by saying 'what what's that' (line 4), he once again establishes himself as lacking knowledge and, given his incorrect terminology, his caseworker fills in the necessary information for the story to continue. The rest of his narrative (lines 6–7) functions to explain how the Individual Living Plan (ILP) works in relation to the expected maximum amount of time a client should be in the shelter. His narrative, however, includes unclear (how does an ILP 'take your place', for example?) and incorrect information. His caseworker provides a dispreferred, or unanticipated and not preferable, response by disagreeing with him ('But').

Here, she begins her own narrative, which also resembles the Labovian structure; however, unlike Labov's stories, this one includes generalised characters, not specific ones. As in earlier extracts, her story begins a pre-sequence that prepares the client for her narrative (which Labov calls an 'abstract') and provides a detailed explanation of the complicating action. Her narrative begins as a story that summarises his extensive stay in the shelter, which she uses to justify her correction of his story (line 17). In line 18, the caseworker slows the phrase 'people started to make this into a home', emphasising the main complicating action in her story. The second part of the narrative establishes a broader institutional frame for understanding both prior and current processes at the shelter. The narrative concludes by stressing the impact of this story on her position at the shelter.

Importantly, the client uses backchannelling devices throughout the entire narrative, but significantly his backchannelling (a device that signals that the caseworker can keep the floor) is simultaneously geared towards maintaining epistemic authority. It takes on an evaluative tone through both the first and the second narrative. Here, the caseworker's narrative functions as an account that seeks to justify why pressure is being placed on the client to find housing and leave the shelter.

Implications for social work practice

This chapter has examined narrative theory and research methods but with a particular orientation to the storytelling occasion rather than seeing the narrative as commenting on the characteristics of the client. Riessman and Quinney (2005) carried out a literature review on narrative in social work and found that the majority of the papers were practice oriented, specifically clinical. They were often case based and explored how clients' stories were addressed therapeutically. There were also examples of self-narratives of client groups. However, they found that narrative theory was rarely applied to the analysis. Overall the authors were disappointed in the research corpus, both the relatively small numbers and the lack of explorations of narrative theory and methods.

Understanding the client

Narrative can offer radically different ways of thinking about the client. The versions of personal and social identity as constructed through narrative provide a major challenge to traditional notions of the individual in social work. Wilks (2005: 1256) provides a strong argument for the significance of narrative ethics that resists the essentialism associated with social work views of people with fixed positions and definable characteristics. Narrative, instead, sees people's identities as becoming, as unfinalised, and moral reasoning as 'narratively shaped'. For Wilks (2005: 1260):

> the idea of moral sensibility [moves] away from the universalism of
> the categorical imperative or pursuit of the good life into a localized,

temporal and changing sphere, much closer to our experience of the moral world.

A number of researchers have investigated the narratives of social work clients, in particular using in-depth interviews as providing a deeper understanding of the client. For example, Wells (2011) analyses the story of a mother whose child was placed in care and then returned home. Martin (1998) describes a project in which young people leaving care were encouraged to tell their stories. In mental illness too, Roe and Davidson (2005: 94) suggest that narrative offers the opportunity to author '"a new story". The process of authoring, in turn, helps consolidate and integrate a sense of self.' While these approaches are important for challenging traditional notions of how social workers understand their clients, we have pointed to some of the limitations of concentrating on interview data and reading through the narrative to the psychology of the storyteller.

Understanding social work practices

Instead, we have promoted an approach to narrative and storytelling that concentrates on the analysis of the storytelling occasion, requiring attention to the audience as much as to the storyteller. Work gets done in storytelling encounters. Clients approach social services agencies often with stories about their problems and how the agency can help. Marvasti (2002) examines how social workers in a homeless agency examine clients' accounts for their 'service-worthiness', by editing the story in terms of the institution's mission.

In our analysis of four narratives told in social worker–client meetings, we have demonstrated how storytelling can serve a number of interactional functions. We saw in Extract 1 how narrative plays a central function in the encounter as the social worker invites stories that structure the encounter and ways of talking about the current state of affairs in the case in particular preferred ways. In Extract 2, the story was used by the client to tell of a key incident to establish ways of formulating the child's progress. In both extracts the social worker assesses the stories in terms of their significance for the case without engaging in the drama of the story. In contrast, in Extracts 3 and 4 the narratives are more contested. In Extract 3 the client tells a story to portray himself as a target, the telling of which the social worker encourages, even if she displays no affiliation. In Extract 4 the social worker and client use competing stories to argue over the appropriate telling of an institutional story.

The reception and subsequent assessment of the story is central to the function of narratives in social work encounters. A number of responses have been identified: the social worker responds to the anxiety of the client in the story; the social worker assesses the story in terms of the current state of the case; the social worker listens to the story but does not acknowledge its significance; and the social worker contests the message of the story. However, in all cases, the social workers have not interrupted the telling of the story, demonstrating the significance of establishing storytelling rights.

Our analysis has concentrated on narrative in encounters between social workers and clients. Other researchers have examined narratives in other social work encounters. Urek (2005) studied how social workers produce stories to produce a particular characterisation of clients to justify decisions and actions through reports and at meetings. Team and supervision meetings are particularly important occasions for the telling of stories. Pithouse and Atkinson (1988) examine how narrative enables the social worker to produce and justify the invisible craftwork of their trade to colleagues and supervisors. Riemann (2005) looks at social work case discussions and, in particular, the balance between narrative and argumentation. He notes how, when social workers describe difficulties in making sense of their cases, the complexity of the stories is lost as colleagues narrow down the evaluation. Crepeau (2000) examines how narratives are told in multi-professional meetings and shows that professionals use stories of particular interactions with services users to evidence their portrayals to colleagues, which is crucial in informing subsequent decision making. This demonstrates the importance of examining narrative and storytelling in all forms of social work encounters.

7

ADVICE-GIVING

Christopher Hall and Stef Slembrouck

Advice-giving in social work is a complex and delicate issue. It is defined by Kadushin and Kadushin (1997: 208) as 'a non-coercive recommendation for some decision or course of action based on professional knowledge'. The social worker is considered to possess knowledge, evidence or judgement that enables the client to access interventions, understand their situation or make choices about their future. A distinction can be made between advice and information: the former involves a 'prescription of a particular course of action for the advice recipient to follow, whereas providing information leaves the decision about what to do to the client' (Kadushin and Kadushin 1997: 208). In the extract below the social worker (SW) responds to the mother's (M) question about support for the cost of a child minder (a provider of day care in their own home while the carer(s) are at work/college) by providing advice.

1	M:	you can help me with child minding because there are two children to pay for and the baby
2	SW:	if you want to go to college yes they can get you child minders
3	M:	alright
4	SW:	but they can't get child minders if you are not doing anything
5	M:	no no no I want [to go to college]
6	SW:	[do you understand me] so if you are going to college there is provision that the
7		college can provide you
8	M:	mm
9	SW:	child minding
10	M:	yeah
11	SW:	ok
12	M:	yeah

13	SW:	that is when you are going if you are not doing anything if you are at home
14	M:	if I go to [particular college]
15	SW:	yeah they will do that they will support you
16	M:	alright
17	SW:	alright
18	M:	that's a good idea

What is noticeable about this extract is that the social worker not only provides information about the availability of child minder support but also advice on the likely qualification for such support (line 4). This extract is advice, not just information, as it is set within a discussion of the benefit to the family of the mother going to college. Importantly, there is a marked acknowledgement (line 18) that the advice has been accepted.

Advice is not always made explicit; a preferred course of action can be implied by the professional (Kadushin and Kadushin 1997: 209). For instance, asking a question or suggesting a different view of a situation seeks to influence the client and is therefore offering advice. It is this location of advice-giving within ongoing social worker–client communication that is the focus of this chapter. Drawing on studies of turn-by-turn interaction, we are interested in both the delivery of advice by the social worker and its reception by the client. However, we are also interested in how advice-giving is linked to wider social work ambitions, for example encouraging clients to cooperate with social work plans.

Advice-giving in the professional literature

In the professional literature, it is often suggested that advice-giving in social work should be kept to a minimum. A social worker may have an investment in providing advice in terms of their construction of the service user's circumstances. This could include explicit direction, something 'should or ought to', which Kadushin and Kadushin note might be 'biased and directs a decision' (1997: 208). Couture and Sutherland (2006: 330) summarise similar concerns in counselling: advice prevents clients from mobilising their own resources; they can become too dependent on the therapist; they may blame the therapist if advice leads to unsatisfactory action; advice is seen as imposing the therapist's value system; and the client might not comply with the advice or might misinterpret it. In summary, advice-giving is seen as a form of social control. In social work, for example, Hollis considers that 'only the beginner or the clumsy worker makes major use of advice' (1964: 94). In a discussion of 'client self-determination', Striker (1990: 226) similarly outlines a case against advice-giving, but then notes: 'In most professions, advice takes the form of a clarification of alternatives and predictions as to possible consequences . . . it can be a way of enabling clients to decide for themselves' (1990: 227). In an older study, Reid and Shapiro (1969) found that even clinical social workers engaged in advice-giving for up to 10 per cent of the time, and moreover service users expected and preferred to receive advice. Concern about advice-giving has led to the development of 'motivational interviewing' in health and social care settings in circumstances where clients display reluctance to change their behaviour, for example regarding substance abuse and smoking. Such a method is contrasted with traditional 'advice-giving' and seen as more effective (Watson 2011: 470).

However, other commentators are less clear that advice-giving can or should be excluded from social work and counselling. Feltham (1995: 18) suggests that counselling is not easily separated from advice-giving; there are occasions when it is 'unethical' to abstain from providing advice. Silverman (1997: 112) notes that 'once we move out of the debate about what is "counselling", it is beyond dispute that advice-giving is a major activity in many professional–client interviews'. Some consumer studies report that clients expect the professional to offer advice (Maluccio 1979). In summary, despite professional reluctance, advice-giving appears to be an inevitable feature of social worker–client interaction. It is important therefore to examine in detail how it is provided, how it is 'heard' (Garfinkel 1967) and how it links to social work ambitions more generally.

Advice-giving in studies of institutional interaction

In social work, advice is treated as an intervention or skill. Having assessed the client's needs, the social worker makes a decision to provide advice, a response selected from a range of possible interventions. However, research that examines professional talk and interaction identifies *advice-giving sequences* as particular forms of interaction or episodes of talk in which features of advice-giving can be identified. The participants might be unaware that advice has been offered or accepted/rejected, in the sense of a deliberate professional move by the social worker or a considered response by the client. Instead, the ongoing interaction between social worker and client results in exchanges that can be identified as advice-giving, with particular features, as well as expectations and obligations on interlocutors that attend to the interactional demands of the current interaction. For instance, Silverman (2000: 144) identifies 'implied advice', which is packaged in questions about the client's personal disposition.

Taking this approach to advice-giving, there are likely to be advice-giving sequences, even in motivational interviewing. In an example examined in Manthey *et al.* (2011), a mother is encouraged to stop taking drugs in order to have her children return home from care. The extract is presented as motivational interviewing as the worker builds on the client's hopes and strengths and avoids 'unsolicited advice' (p. 144). However, when we examine the interaction as a whole, it can nevertheless be seen as an advice-giving sequence, since the worker encourages the mother to see that her hopes for her children to return home involve addressing her drug abuse:

Worker:	So the biggest barrier to you achieving the goal of having custody of your kids is drug use. (Reflection)
Julie:	Yes, they told me that as long as I was using I couldn't keep my kids.
Worker:	And you really want your kids back because being a mother is a big part of who you are as a person, you love your kids, and you think you would be good at taking care of your kids. (Reflection)
Julie:	Yeah, I would be good at taking care of my kids. No one else should parent my kids. I'm a good mom.
Worker:	Having your kids live with you would be the best thing for your kids. (Reflection).
Julie:	Yes! They tell me they want to come back and live with me and they miss me so much. I love my sister, but she isn't their mother. I am their mother and I know them best and how to take care of them best.

(Manthey *et al.* 2011: 140)

In the extract above the worker's comments are coded as 'reflections'; however, these turns are responded to by the client as if they are 'questions'. Crucially, they are questions that solicit preferred answers and imply desired courses of action. The comment 'having your kids live with you would be the best thing for your kids' is stating a preferred position, which inter-actionally invites an agreement. While this is not an explicit instance of unsolicited advice, the sequence as a whole can be seen as advice-giving.

In a study of advice-giving by health visitors Heritage and Sefi (1992: 368) suggest that advice-giving can be analysed in terms of 'sequences in which the health visitor describes, recommends or otherwise forwards a preferred course of future action'. They highlight three types: 'overt recommendations', for example 'Well my advice to you is that . . .'; advice couched in the imperative mood, for example 'always be very very quiet at night'; and the use of verbs that express obligation, for example 'and I think you should involve your husband as much as possible'. Silverman (1997: 111) sees aids counselling as organised to promote preferred courses of action rather than merely providing information for the patient to use as they wish.

Gillespie and Cornish (2010) note in a study of health visitors that 'giving advice is not simply presenting new knowledge, rather it re-positions the advice-giver and advice receiver with complex consequences'. Vehviläinen (2001: 373) notes that 'in counselling, which involves a strong orientation to the clients' autonomy . . . and to the obligation to respect the client's experience, advice giving requires particular interactional work on the part of the adviser'. Butler *et al.* (2010) note two important interactional characteristics of advice-giving. It is *normative* as it implies a preferred course of action that the recipient should undertake. It is also *asymmetric* as the advice-giver is positioned as more knowledgeable than the recipient.

Research that examines advice-giving in health and social care has been the subject of some of the key texts in the analysis of institutional talk and interaction (e.g. Heritage and Sefi 1992; Jefferson and Lee 1992; Silverman 1997). In such work, advice-giving is seen as an inevitable feature of professional practices. Furthermore, as with the professional literature, the potential interactional dilemmas associated with advice-giving are identified in studies of talk and interaction in institutional encounters. Jefferson and Lee (1992: 531) suggest that 'acceptance or rejection [of advice] may be in great part an interactional matter, produced by reference to the current talk, more or less independent of intention to use it, or actual subsequent use'. The implications of this approach are that a social worker might be providing appropriate advice, but because of the timing of the formulation and the sequence of interaction in which it occurs, the advice is treated as interactionally inappropriate, and it is resisted or ignored by the client.

Studies of talk and interaction in professional practices have examined advice-giving across health and social care services – for example, health visitors (Heritage and Sefi 1992), HIV counselling (Silverman 1997), telephone support lines (Pudlinski 2002), GPs (Pilnick and Coleman 2003) and social workers (Suoninen and Jokinen 2005). We will now discuss these studies in detail, especially those by Heritage and colleagues.

Advice-giving by health visitors

As a contrast to social work, we will examine the detailed analysis of advice-giving by health visitors to new mothers by Heritage and colleagues (Heritage and Sefi 1992; Heritage and Lindström 2012). They note the potential interactional difficulties. The mothers treated the health visitors as 'baby experts' rather than 'befrienders'. The health visitor may also be seen as someone who 'stands in judgement on the mother's competence in child care [which] suggests that requesting and giving advice during these first visits can be highly problematic activities' (Heritage and Sefi 1992: 367). The mothers might see their own knowledge and competence as an object of evaluation (Heritage and Sefi 1992: 366). The authors provide an example of an exchange where the health visitor comments on the baby's sucking behaviour:

> HV: He's enjoying that [isn't he
> F: [Yes he certainly is
> M: He's not hungry cos he's just had his bottle
>   (Heritage and Sefi 1992: 367; transcription simplified)

The father takes the remark at face value, whereas the mother interprets the comment as saying that the baby might be hungry and hence as a potential criticism.

In their corpus, few of the advice-giving sequences were initiated by the mothers (Heritage and Sefi 1992: 376); more often they were initiated by the health visitors, mainly from routine enquiries about the babies and the mothers' health. Heritage and Sefi (1992: 377) describe the interactional problem for the health visitor as establishing collaboration with the mother and constructing a context in which advice is offered in an appropriate way. They identify a sequence that they describe as 'stepwise entry in the advice-giving', in which the health visitor and mother can jointly identify a problem and thereafter facilitate an acceptable move to advice-giving.

In the first step the health visitor enquires about a potentially difficult matter. The mother responds that there have been some problematic aspects. The health visitor asks more questions about the problem to which the mother provides more detail. Finally the advice is given. An example they provide concerns the baby's cord:

```
HV:   is the cord ehm (1) dry now
M:    Yes it's (.) it weeps a little bit
HV:   and what do you do[
M:                        [m'yeah I've some of these mediswabs
HV:   [uh huh
M:    [an' I use it to clean it with and I put a bit of talcum powder
      on
HV:   don't be frightened of the cord. . . .
```
(Heritage and Sefi 1992: 377–379;
transcription simplified)

In the third turn the health visitor establishes the issue as problematic and requiring action, and asks for more information to make way for a solution. Note how the advice starts with a state of mind, 'don't be frightened', before providing detailed advice. Heritage and Sefi (1992: 380) argue that such a sequence establishes the relevance and need for advice, which is provided in non-adversarial fashion. However, they add that the majority of the encounters did not follow such a sequence; the health visitor usually moved to advice before a problem had been established or before it had been assessed if advice would be welcomed.

Heritage and colleagues also examined the responses of the mothers to advice-giving, which they describe as marked acknowledgement, unmarked acknowledgement and assertions of knowledge and competence. In the case of marked acknowledgements, the mother reacts to the advice with an explicit response, for example 'oh right', which both establishes the advice as 'news' and suggests acceptance. In these exchanges the mother has already cast herself as a 'prospective advice recipient' (Heritage and Sefi 1992: 395). In unmarked acknowledgements, in contrast, the mother responds to the advice with 'continuers' such as 'mm, yeah', which do not treat the advice as 'news' nor acknowledge the talk as advice. They often move to a different topic rather than treat the talk as advice. Heritage and Sefi (1992: 396) see such reactions as 'passive resistance' (see Chapter 8 on resistance). Assertions of knowledge also display resistance to advice, as mothers show their competence ('I know') and treat the advice as not news. Despite displays of knowledge, Heritage and Sefi (1992: 409) note that the health visitors continue their advice-giving and thereby 'sequentially delete the mothers' claims to competence'. In a later paper, Heritage and Lindström (2012) note that the health visitor prolongs the advice-giving in the hope of marked uptakes, with resulting interaction difficulties as to how the topic can be closed. Overall, Heritage and Sefi (1992: 410) estimate that three-quarters of health visitor-initiated advice was met with passive or active resistance.

Heritage and colleagues' research provided an important foundation for studying advice-giving in professional–client exchanges and will be used as a contrast throughout this chapter, since social workers, like health visitors, are seen as having a surveillance role, though with different statutory and regulatory responsibilities. Heritage and Sefi (1992: 411) note the 'clinical problem-oriented approach of health visiting', which is contrasted with 'those whose training originates in social work'. However, they also note that less initiated advice was offered when the same health visitors were talking to experienced mothers. So both the context and the experience of the professional have an impact on how advice is offered.

Advice-giving in other health and social care settings

Silverman (1997) analyses advice-giving in HIV counselling, and found similar practices to those identified by Heritage and colleagues. Here, the counsellor is obligated to provide health education messages as part of their work to support the patient as they await the results of the HIV test. The counselling 'simply comes along with getting an HIV test rather than "help" requested by the client' (Silverman 1997: 113). Silverman makes an important distinction between an 'information delivery format' and an 'interview format'. In the former, advice is not personalised to the patient's perspective and it is often delivered without the patient having identified a perceived problem. This often results in minimal acknowledgement, but tends not to result in overt rejection. In the interview format, by contrast, advice-giving is delayed until the patient perspective has been elicited, enabling the counsellor to tailor the advice to what the client has revealed (p. 117). However, personalised advice-giving requires stronger uptake, and it is hard for the client to ignore. While these are quite different approaches, they are often used interchangeably. Like Heritage and colleagues, Silverman (1997:

126–127) found that advice was mostly initiated by the counsellor and most acknowledgements were unmarked. Resistance tended to emerge 'where a counsellor embarks on a piece of advice that has not been grounded first in her client's own perspective' (Silverman 1997: 152), echoing Heritage and Sefi.

Leppänen (1998) compared advice-giving by district nurses in Sweden with the sequences described by Heritage and Sefi. He found far fewer examples of advice-giving and few used the stepwise approaches described above. This is explained by district nurses providing specific tests or treatments to patients and the advice-giving being 'simply a consequence of incidental observations of problems' (p. 234). Furthermore, district nurses met 'experienced patients', suggesting that advice was not an expected feature of the encounter.

Pilnick and Coleman (2003) analysed the ways in which GPs offer advice about smoking cessation. These were routine consultations about the patient's health, in which the GP topicalised smoking cessation as a preferred course of action to address the patient's condition. The authors identify less direct forms, in addition to instances in which advice occurs in the form of direct instructions. In some instances, smoking is presented as 'a general problem for people in a particular circumstance':

GP:	The people they are saying should change are those who are overweight, smoke or have a history of thrombosis in the close family ... for now if you don't fit into any of these categories ...
Patient:	Well I smoke
GP:	Yes
Patient:	Fifteen a day
GP:	(pause) I think then that probably should put you into that category where you should think of changing.

(Pilnick and Coleman 2003: 138)

The advice is offered after the patient has placed themselves in one of the vulnerable groups that the GP has identified. It has an indirect manner and hence is less threatening. Pilnick and Coleman also analyse a situation that they term 'worst case scenario', where the GP affirms that stopping smoking is the solution to the problem, and meets strong resistance from the patient.

In social work, Suoninen and Jokinen (2005) look at advice-giving in terms of the ways in which social workers persuade clients to cooperate with preferred actions. As with the comments above, they note that direct advice-giving may come with a risk of threatening face, so more indirect ways are examined. They discuss 'persuasive questions' in which the respondent is given 'the power to state how things are. A social worker as an interviewer, however, may include some "hints" about adequate answers in her questions' (Suoninen and Jokinen 2005: 471). They provide an example of a social worker discussing with a mother her children's lateness for school. After several attempts to raise the issue, the social worker provides a candidate solution that the children could 'have an alarm clock of their own'. Suoninen and Jokinen (2005: 464) comment:

> The social worker does not give clear-cut advice e.g. by saying 'you must resolve this problem'. However she hints at such an obligation by asking 'have you now done that', 'so what have you done about this matter' and in the end 'could the boys have an alarm clock of their own?'

The authors also note that the mother does not take 'a position of a recipient of advice' in the first two interactions, and even in the third 'she minimizes the effect of the advice'. These studies suggest that there are complex versions of advice-giving, often associated with the advice-giver being sensitive to the dangers of rejection by the advice recipient. Advice is often provided indirectly, sometimes after the client's perspective has been elicited, and it can be part of a general feature of affiliation and persuasion in professional–service user interaction.

Couture and Sutherland (2006) provide a detailed analysis of an advice-giving sequence in family therapy, building on the stepwise approach of Heritage and Sefi. The therapist offers a topic for consideration, in this case how the conflict between a young person and his parents might be resolved. The therapist assesses the extent to which the parents have accepted that the topic needs to be considered and then offers advice. In the extract, the therapist asks how long the parents think the contract by the young person to be involved in therapy will last. The parents comment that they had not considered this. The therapist adds that the young person should have the opportunity to renegotiate the arrangement. The parents agree that the contract will not last forever. The researchers' detailed analysis of this sequence raises the relevance of a number of specific interactional features. The therapist uses the topic management marker, 'ok', to flag a new topic for consideration. The question itself is introduced with various hesitations, which contribute to building up a sense of curiosity. Humour is used to undermine the position that the contract should not be reviewed. The authority of the advice is offered cautiously and downgraded to a suggestion (rather than an opinion) by the use of 'I think'. As Couture and Sutherland (2006) summarise, 'this stance of "talking to listen" facilitates a collaborative, forward-moving process ... active participants rather than passive opinion recipients' (p. 337). The interaction builds on careful negotiations to establish explicitly constructed agreements with the participants.

This review of the literature has concentrated on studies of advice-giving developed over sequences and their interactional accomplishment. Discourse analytic approaches often treat advice-giving as an example of an adjacency pair, consisting of 'advice offer' and 'advice accept/reject' (Sacks *et al.* 1974). The sequential orientation also highlights implied advice, where the advice is accomplished by asking questions that imply preferred answers. We wish to argue that an exclusively formal-functional treatment, though considerably enriched by the identification of alternative patterns and variations within these, might still be too restrictive in scope. In attempting to understand professional–client talk as accomplishing professional practice, it seems we need to extend the idea of advice-giving sequences, so as to accord it a place within professional practice more generally. This means linking the analysis of advice-giving in actual exchanges with concepts associated with the profession of social work, for example the achievement of professional goals, versions of clients and their preferred/dispreferred characteristics, and generic principles of how to talk and conceptualise social and personal problems. Advice-giving in professional encounters therefore is concerned not merely with the place in the sequences but also with the accomplishment of professional practice. It requires identifying more than a particular type of turn-pair, as Locher and Limberg (2012: 3) comment: not only the speech act but 'attempting to grasp the practice of advice-seeking and advice-giving more globally, the speech activity'.

Advice-giving in social work interaction: data examples and analyses

We will now examine three advice-giving sequences and make some suggestions as to how they can be analysed. We are particularly interested in developing concepts identified by Heritage and colleagues, notably how advice is prepared for, offered and received. However, we are also interested in how social worker–client encounters involve the negotiation of advice that is consequential for ongoing social work, rather than advice on a non-personal, 'take it or leave it' basis. The data extracts are from various social work settings in the UK and were collected as part of a research project to examine professional–client communication in collaboration with social workers (Hall *et al.* 2010; Slembrouck and Hall 2011).

Advice is offered and received

In this case the social worker has been visiting the family for several months as part of a child protection plan. The mother had been the subject of a serious domestic assault and she and her children had been rehoused from a different part of the city to escape the father. The social worker is providing support with this relocation as well as ensuring the safety of the family. The first topic to be raised during the home visit is an update on repairs to the heating in the home. The social worker enquires how the family is coping with the lack of heating. It is December and quite cold.

Extract 1

1	SW:	ok that's fine erm so I saw one heater there
2	M:	[yeah]
3	SW:	[have] you got any other heater in here
4	M:	I have another one similar like this in the kitchen
5	SW:	in the kitchen
6	M:	yeah
7	SW:	so how are the children coping with the heating
8	M:	well what we do is erm this one and the two they gave me
9	SW:	yes
10	M:	I bought one extra one which is three
11	SW:	ok making three
12	M:	yeah so I gave one to ((child's name)) and ((child's name))
13	SW:	very [good]
14	M:	[one] to the two boys' bedroom
15	SW:	very good
16	M:	one for me and the [two children]
17	SW:	[and the two children] making three so you are happy with that
18	M:	[well we just surviving]
19	SW:	[it's managing]
20	M:	as soon as it's snowing you know
21	SW:	ok
22	M:	freezing
23	SW:	ok so I will advise you to phone them later today (.) that the place is freezing (.) that they
24		should assist you to come and do the job proper quickly. I will also when I get back to work I
25		will send an email
26	M:	hhuh
27	SW:	to housing repairs to come out and do something for us as I'm here now it's slightly cold
28	M:	yeah it is it's very
29	SW:	ok
30	M:	I told them yesterday that I got six children and you know I got a baby here and it's not
31	SW:	exactly
32	M:	it's not good because we then have what you call a cold wind no hot water it's
33	SW:	mhm
34	M:	difficult for me to wash the dishes and cook it's freezing the water you know
35	SW:	ok
36	M:	I can't touch it and you know the children they can't use the water
37	SW:	ok
38	M:	every time I have to warm it through the cooker and then give it to them which is very very
39		difficult
40	SW:	difficult ok
41	M:	yeah [so]
42	SW	[I will] look into that I will I will it would be very good if you can contact them

43		[and also]
44	M:	[I I contacted them] yesterday and I'm going to call them today as well
45	SW:	please
46	M:	yes definitely [because]
47	SW:	[alright] (2) now that is that now apart from that have you any health problems

Before this extract, the topic of the lack of heating is raised by the social worker. In response, the mother provides a report on the progress of the repairs. The social worker now focuses on the impact on the family by asking about the number of temporary heaters that have been provided and which the mother details in lines 4–16. This topic is introduced with the comment 'I saw one heater' (line 1), and aims to explore how the problem is experienced by the family: 'how are the children coping' (line 7). This focusing in on the problem moves the discussion from the general (the work is being held up) to the specific (the current heating of the home). It is formulated in terms of a potential problem for the children, in line with the social worker's child-focused remit. After the report by the mother, the social worker does not provide an assessment but asks if this is adequate: 'so you are happy with that' (line 17). That question is framed as a potential closing remark, the current heating is adequate, suggesting that the situation is not so problematic. However, the mother resists this formulation: 'we [are] just surviving' (line 18), which the social worker downgrades to 'managing' (line 19). The mother again resists the formulation and upgrades the problem: 'it's snowing you know' (line 20) and 'freezing' (line 22).

The social worker now provides advice about contacting the housing department immediately. This is strongly formulated in the form of a three-item list with pauses between each clause: 'phone them later today', 'the place is freezing', 'they should assist ... and do the job proper'. The list identifies the action, the current problem and who is responsible. The shared nature of the problem is also highlighted in line 27: 'do something for us' and 'as I'm here now it's slightly cold' (although the extent of the problem is downgraded from freezing to slightly cold). The mother does not acknowledge the advice and indeed responds that she has already contacted them (line 30), treating the advice as redundant. She now highlights the implications for the children of 'no hot water' (lines 32 to 39). The social worker concurs with the situation being 'difficult' (line 40), in contrast to the mother's 'very very difficult' (lines 38–39). He then reiterates the advice at line 42 but first hints at his action and then stresses the importance of her action. The mother repeats that she contacted them yesterday but agrees to do so again (line 44). The social worker asks explicitly 'please' (line 45) and the mother concurs, more strongly now: 'yes definitely'. She appears to want to continue the discussion with 'because' (line 46), but the social worker closes the topic: 'alright now that is that' (line 47).

If we go back to Heritage and Sefi's (1992) stepwise entry into advice-giving, we can detect the five stages in the excerpt above – social worker raises the potential problem (is there enough heating?), the mother confirms the problem (not enough heaters), the enquiry is focused (are these heaters enough?), and there is responsive detailing (just surviving, freezing) and advice (phone the housing department). However, the reception of the advice is not straightforward. The mother appears initially to reject the advice: she extends the problem and only agrees to the action after a specific request. Even then, she appears to try to extend the discussion. Throughout the inter-action, the mother's and the social worker's evaluations of the seriousness of the problem have been slightly at odds with each other. Perhaps, if the advice had contained more 'news' as Heritage and Sefi suggest, for example suggestions of a particular housing officer to approach or instructions on how the complaint might be better framed, the mother might have appeared more satisfied. In terms of the social work task, the advice-giving has been directive, even imploring ('please' line 45) and it has been accepted with agreement for a joint and coordinated action. However, given the way in which the social worker closes the sequence, the advice comes across more like a response to a spate of troubles-telling (Jefferson and Lee 1992) than as an intervention aimed at, for example, advice on how to make complaints.

Advice is offered, but not acknowledged

The second extract is from a home visit by a family support worker (FSW) to a mother (M) who has a three-year-old child with autism (J). The profes-sional has been working with the mother for several months and considered that she had developed a good relationship, providing support to the mother to promote her care of her child and the child's learning and development. A feature of the ongoing work was that the professional was careful to divide her attention equally between the needs of the mother and those of the child. In the sequence below the advice-giving relates to a suggestion at an earlier meeting that the mother should consider having a genetic test. The advice is expert advice, in the sense that it is embedded in expert knowledge about population probabilities. At the same time we see a case-specific feature of the advice-giving emerge – whether to have another baby. The topic was developed from a discussion initiated by the mother about a recent TV programme in which a family had three children with autism. The professional uses the opportunity to transform the talk into advice-giving.

Extract 2

1	M:	((partner)) was the one watching the news
2	FSW:	oh on the national autistic day. So what did he talk about then
3	M:	he was just telling me he was not alone there was others out there as well like he told me about

4		he saw this lady on the TV with three children ((with autism))
5	FSW:	like we were saying in that meeting there is a tendency ehm for it ((autism)) to run in families
6		Sometimes you can have one autistic child ehm and your other children will be fine but other
7		times it does it can run in the family so that's why we were talking about getting you tested
8		and things to see whether that's likely or not ehm (.) you yeah imagine to have three children
9		it would be hard
10	M:	I'd commit suicide straight away
11	FSW:	ah but you've done so well with J though. Maybe you'll be an expert by then
12	M:	no I couldn't go through it again. It's scarin' me now. I'm scared to have another child
13	FSW:	yeah
14	M:	I'm going to take my time
15	FSW:	yeah well you've still got plenty of time to decide ehm but you should definitely think about
16		the testing. That will you give you an idea and will help you make up your mind
17	M:	yeah
18	FSW:	y'know and even if you didn't want to have another baby of your own you can think about
19		other options that you could do
20	M:	I want to foster
21	FSW:	I thought you might
22	M:	definitely. I always said that. No matter what job I find, I'm going to end up fostering.
23	FSW:	that's a really nice thing to do and ehm so yeah, it doesn't close all the doors for you y'know
24		if the news weren't to be the best news. There's lots of other things that you can still do. So
25	M:	[to child] sorry baba. Did that go in your eye? Are you playing with me
26	FSW:	(laughs) so yeah

In this extract, the construction of an advice-giving sequence builds upon the mother's initiation of the topic, a family where there were three children with autism. Initially this is not necessarily raised as a problematic matter, rather a report that other families have the problems we have, only more so. It is reassuring; the father constructs himself as 'not alone' (line 3), using an upgraded contrast: our own difficult situation *versus* a much more complex one. The FSW moves to construct this as a problem, 'autism runs in families' (line 5) and, in doing so, proceeds from a general to the more personal situation of this family: 'getting you tested and things' (lines 7–8). The pause on line 8 by the FSW invites the mother to acknowledge the advice immediately. However, without such uptake, the FSW explores the problem further: 'imagine to have three children it would be hard' (lines 8–9). The problem elaboration occurs after the advice.

The mother responds to the problem with an extreme case formulation (Pomerantz 1986): 'I'd commit suicide' (line 10); such a situation is unthinkable. The FSW attempts to reduce such a formulation and at the same time depicts the mother as a potential expert (line 11). However, in response the mother maintains her strong reaction to the situation with a three-part formulation: 'couldn't go through it again', 'scarin' me now', 'I'm scared to have another child' (line 12). This is a particularly strong rhetorical feature, which defines and upgrades the problem: having another child with autism. This statement is much stronger than the depiction of the potential problem by the FSW in line 9. The FSW merely acknowledges the mother's strong formulation 'yeah' (line 13), with neither support nor criticism and the mother reduces the high anxiety of the previous formulation from 'I'm scared' to 'I'm going to take my time' (line 14). In lines 15–16 the FSW concurs with the mother about taking time but repeats the advice. This version of the advice is more emphatic, 'definitely think about the testing', with added justification: this may 'help you make up your mind'. The mother provides only minimal acknowledgement of the advice 'yeah' (line 17). The FSW extends the justification for the advice, to enable consideration of other options (line 19), which the mother takes as an opportunity to introduce a topic change: 'fostering' (line 20). Lines 21 and 22 attend to this new topic, and although the FSW offers more advantages of testing: 'if the news weren't to be the best news. There's lots of other things that you can still do' (line 24), the mother turns her attention to the child (line 25), which the FSW accepts, 'so yeah' (line 26). The topic is closed.

Compared to Heritage and Sefi's formulation, this advice about getting tested has not been offered in a stepwise entry. It is not responded to as 'news' since it had been raised at a previous meeting. Most importantly, there is no 'marked acknowledgement' by the mother, only a minimal 'yeah' (line 17) followed by a topic change. We cannot identify from this exchange any agreement by the mother with the advice to 'get herself tested'. However, is there any evidence in this exchange that the mother has seen this as unwelcome advice or has she displayed 'passive resistance', as Heritage and colleagues might suggest? The next section of the home visit becomes a very sensitive discussion about the nature of autism, whether the mother's genes are to blame and whether other members of her family might be autistic. The advice of being tested is not raised again. The FSW does not produce a stronger invitation to pursue the advice, for example 'so shall I make an appointment for you'. Instead, the topic is on the table, available to be revisited in the future. We might suggest, therefore, that the advice is not unwelcome but nor is it accepted. Advice-giving here is an element in the ongoing negotiation of appropriate action between FSW and mother in an ongoing relationship. That the advice is not accepted explicitly at this point does not suggest that it will not continue to be introduced on other occasions and perhaps it becomes an action point in a future care plan.

Advice after establishing affiliation

The next extract is taken from an interview with a mother (M) whose daughter has recently returned home from care, aged 18. The social worker (SW) has supported the family in this process but is also involved because of previous domestic violence. The opening exchanges have focused on the difficulties that have occurred with the daughter returning to the home, the limited space in the flat and her lack of a job or training. The sequence is different from those above in that the advice-giving is aimed at suggesting how the mother should think about the daughter rather than merely recommending specific action.

Extract 3

1	SW:	((service user's name)) one more thing that I I would like you to mention don't take it
2		personally but what what happens sometimes when children have seen a lot during their
3		childhood, for example there was
4	M:	[yeah]
5	SW:	[a lot of a difficult period when they went into care
6	M:	yes
7	SW:	when you were quite a lot, it was difficult for you to leave alcohol and you were quite quite
8		used to using alcohol and abusing it and [husband], that's
9	M:	[yeah]
10	SW:	((child's name)) and ((child's name)) father, he was also doing the same thing and then he was
11		obviously there was a lot of domestic violence on yourself
12	M:	yes
13	SW:	and you suffered a lot so I think you were you were trying to you can say that you were
14		trying to umm umm (.) decrease it in a way by using alcohol and just
15	M:	[yeah]
16	SW:	just assuming that everything is fine
17	M:	I felt I was treading water basically I wasn't getting anywhere [at that point it was dreadful]
18	SW:	[anywhere you were going in circles
19	M:	yes
20	SW:	and it is it is it's you can say that we we have backed it with research that sometimes this
21		happens with children also when because they have seen this in their childhood
22	M:	yes
23	SW:	it comes back to them and they and it's not fair to say that she she had a normal childhood
24		it's not fair
25	M:	[no] the more and more the more and more I realise actually the further away it gets the
26		more I'm looking at her and realise just how how devastating the the that alcoholism has
27		been in her she
28	SW:	mmm
29	M:	isn't like a what I would categorise as a normal teenager who she's not she's a damaged
30		child [and I]
31	SW:	[yeah] she she she is a a damaged child
32	M:	I have to put that into perspective I have to try and [think] about that you know like be
33	SW:	[yeah]
34	M:	and be sympathetic about it
35	SW:	that's what that's what I was saying to you when you were saying no she's not allowed I was

36		saying that I understand where you are coming from but at the same time this is not all her
37		fault
38	M:	no no it isn't
39	SW:	it it it can be, I'm not saying that it's your fault totally but at the same time obviously you
40		were the [adults] in her life
41	M:	[yeah]
42	SW:	and she was a child at that time. But it's it's good that she has agreed for joint counselling I
43		think that's a brilliant idea
44	M:	yep it is
45	SW:	um it's good, so when she is more settled she can look at going to the job centre . . .

Immediately before this extract the mother had reported how, although things were difficult, she would try her best to help her daughter settle back at home and find a job or training. While these sentiments are supported by the social worker, this sequence is premised on the basis that the mother also needs to adjust her thinking about the child. The beginning displays marked hedging as the social worker addresses the mother by her Christian name and appeals to a generalisation ('what happens sometimes when children have seen a lot', line 2) and a disclaimer ('don't take it personally', lines 1–2), clearly alerting the mother to the sensitivity of what is to follow. The appeal to a generalisation, 'what is typical for people in your situation', is a classic face-mitigating device and typical of 'advice as information' sequences (Heritage and Lindström 2012). The social worker provides a long explanation of difficulties that children in general and this child in particular have faced when living with parents who abuse alcohol and where there is domestic violence (lines 7–16). This is a long turn with few occasions available for the mother to respond; there is a strong display of expertise on child development. Only at lines 6 and 12 is there enough of a pause for her to display agreement. At line 17 the mother displays a strong affiliation with the social worker's formulation, 'I felt I was treading water basically I wasn't getting anywhere', but this agreement is treated as an interruption and the social worker continues with general formulations about the effects on children 'backed by research' (line 20).

At line 23 the social worker contends that the daughter has not had a 'normal childhood'. This formulation is immediately accepted by the mother at lines 25–27. Her turn is hurried, repeating 'more and more', 'the the' and 'realise'. She repeats the social worker's view that her daughter is not a normal child but transforms this into the category of a 'damaged child' (line 29). The social worker immediately agrees with this formulation. These are strong affiliations around serious subjects. The category of a 'damaged child' opens the possibility of strong self-blaming by the mother. The agreement has been very carefully worked up by the social worker but without allowing room for the 'problem-indicative responses' and 'responsive detailing' that Heritage and Sefi identify. It is similar to Couture and Sutherland's idea of identifying a 'shared middle ground' (2006: 337) between a troubled teenager and bewildered parents – the construction of a formulation that the young person's behaviour is understandable given what has happened to them. They see such a process as similar to the 'stepwise entry into advice', as the therapist attempts to reach an agreement with the parents on how the problem is to be understood.

When there is agreement on the problem, then advice can be provided. In this case the social worker relies on the agreed characterisation of a 'damaged child' to formulate a criticism of the mother's actions: 'that's what I was saying to you when you were saying no she's not allowed, I was saying ... this is not all her fault' (lines 35–37). Again the mother displays agreement (line 38). From line 42 onwards, the social worker is now able to provide advice on specific action: 'joint counselling is a brilliant idea' and 'when she is more settled she can look at going to the job centre' (line 45).

In this extract, the social worker takes a problem identified by the client, the child returning home, and reformulates it, drawing on expert formulations. The mother is persuaded to think more sympathetically about her daughter: given the previous history, the mother's own behaviour is implicated in the child's behaviour. The mother agrees with the formulation and displays strong affiliation by providing a category, 'a damaged child'. Such collaborative categorisation work (Hall *et al.* 2006) acts as a necessary precursor to advice on appropriate action: counselling, finding a job. In contrast to Extracts 1 and 2, the social worker's ambition here is one of attitude change. It is central to the interaction and agreements are necessary before action can be supported. In this case, advice on action can be supported once the social worker and mother share an appropriate understanding of the child's behaviour.

Implications for social work practice

We have seen in this chapter that advice-giving and its reception is often a central dilemma in professional–client interaction. It is also an arena in which managing resistance is a feature, although resistance in these extracts has been passive (Extract 2). Hepburn and Potter (2011: 218) note that displays of competence by advice receivers (as in Extracts 1 and 3) might be seen as affiliation rather than resistance (see Chapter 8 on resistance). The professional social work literature has often suggested that advice-giving should be avoided because it would be associated with bad practice. In our corpus of 22 social worker–client meetings, we identified between four and 24 advice-giving sequences per meeting, whereas Heritage and Sefi found 70 in eight home visits (1992: 360). Why might this be? Are these extracts examples of poor practice?

As the discourse analytic literature shows, advice-giving is a ubiquitous feature of both everyday and institutional interaction. Advice-giving sequences are features of encounters in which people talk about their troubles, seek solutions or are perceived as seeking solutions. Social work is one such occasion, albeit one with expectations as to whose troubles are the subject of the talk. Seen in this way, advice-giving is not necessarily formulated as a chosen professional intervention. Some examples of advice-giving are therefore more mundane and emerge in social worker–client talk in which everyday troubles are discussed, as in Extract 1 (contacting the housing office). The social worker has an expertise to suggest options for resolving everyday problems – access services, handle children's behaviour, manage household tasks and so on.

Other instances of advice-giving are more closely linked to social work ambitions more generally, as we saw in Extract 2: advice to help the client address particular dilemmas (to have a genetic test to help decide on having another child) and Extract 3, advice to persuade the client to change attitudes (to think differently about her child). The social worker's advice is part of ongoing discussions and negotiations, of which this particular sequence is an instance. Similar advice might have been offered on previous occasions (as noted in Extract 2) and the advice is not necessarily offered and accepted; it may be revisited later and reformulated. Advice-giving is part of establishing agreements in ongoing social work. The social worker might in these instances deliberately raise topics to revisit and re-enforce previous advice but not necessarily expect immediate or sustained uptake. Notably the advice-giving did not follow the steps suggested by Heritage and colleagues, primarily because it is not news. However, in both cases the social worker attended to the delicacy of the topic. In Extract 2, agreement to have a genetic test was not sought but left up in the air as an option. In Extract 3, diverting blame from the child to the mother was managed with considerable delicacy.

In summary, we have demonstrated the importance of advice-giving in social work talk. However, we have suggested that both the social work literature and the discourse analytic literature need to be revised. The social work literature needs to see advice-giving as an inevitable feature of troubles-telling encounters and as interactional work. The discourse analytic literature needs to see that advice-giving in social work is more than a speech act or limited to a set of two turns; it is part of the longer-term establishing of agreements and ways of thinking. If advice-giving is seen as a link between mundane professional–client interaction and professional ambitions, then it is an important concept for our understanding of social work practices.

8

RESISTANCE

Kirsi Juhila, Dorte Caswell and Suvi Raitakari

Resistance is a well-recognised phenomenon in social work. The prevailing way to understand it in professional social work discourse is to focus on clients' reactions and behaviour. As Miller (2003: 193) states, professionals tend to 'discuss troubles in their relationships with clients as evidence of client resistance'. So, it is generally assumed by social workers that clients and professionals divide into two *confrontational camps*, due to resistance on the part of the client. The most obvious professional explanation for this confrontation is that clients do not behave like professionals expect them to behave: they resist acknowledging their problems and thus they also resist change, and they do not follow professionals' advice, recommendations and so on (Miller 2003). This kind of resistance is often regarded as clients' normal responses in ambivalent situations, and the professionals' task and even responsibility is to work with it and, in the end, manage it using, for instance, motivational interviewing (Watson 2011). This line of reasoning is clearly built in to some professional theories, such as cognitive self-change programmes or psychoanalytically oriented approaches (Fox 2001; Vehviläinen 2008). What is almost unnoticed and silenced in this under-standing of resistance is the social workers' own resistance. When clients as individual actors are categorised as resistant persons, the professionals' resistance, for instance towards clients' interpretations of their problems or towards their refusal of offered services, can be easily bypassed.

In addition to this dominant view of seeing resistance as confrontations between clients and social workers caused by resistant clients, there is another way to approach resistance in social work discourse. That is to see social workers and clients more as *allies*, being in the same boat, jointly resisting oppressive and inequality-producing societal structures, ideologies and labelling. Instead of categorising resistant clients as 'non-behaving', they are defined as strong and empowered with a right to advocate for themselves. This understanding of resistance is what we often call critical or anti-discriminatory social work practice (e.g. Payne 1997; Adams *et al.* 2002; Barnes and Prior 2009).

Resistance as a research topic has received increasing attention in the social sciences in recent decades. However, there is no consensus about what phenomena and actions fill the criteria of resistance. Instead of an agreed definition there are various understandings, which share a view that emphasis on resistance means a move away from researching inflexible social structures and top-down social control towards the issues of agencies and practices (Hollander and Einwohner 2004). Acts of resistance are something that are produced and created in 'here and now' local practices. They are neither simple reactions to repressive power and control nor intentional acts conducted independently by other actors (Thomas and Davies 2005). Following this emphasis we examine and illustrate in this chapter how resistance can be studied as accomplishments in interaction in social work settings. We include a focus on ways in which resistance can be produced by both clients and social workers. We discuss resistance both as confrontations between clients and workers and as resistance against common enemies, and show what interactional studies add to these two discourses of resistance. We also wish to demonstrate that whether resistance is to be understood as a positive or a negative force in social work depends on members' – social workers' as well as clients' – orientations.

How resistance is displayed and what is resisted in social work interaction

In previous literature on social work and related professional interaction, resistance has been studied as local accomplishments from multiple angles. We have classified this multiplicity into three lines of research: (1) resistance as sequential actions, (2) resistance towards stigmatised categorisations, and (3) resistance towards institutional and governmental policies. The first line of research – resistance as sequential actions – focuses on studying turn-by-turn interaction and analyses how resistance can be located in it. The direction of research unfolds from 'how questions' (resistant turns of talk as sequential phenomena) to 'what questions' (what is resisted with resistant turns). The other two follow mainly the opposite direction, starting from 'what questions' (what categorisations, what policies) and proceeding to 'how questions' (ways categorisations and policies are resisted). In social work interaction, all these 'what and how' actions can be present within each conversation. We illustrate this simultaneous presence through data examples that follow the literature review.

Resistance as sequential actions

Resistance as sequential actions in professional–client interaction is a well-researched area, especially in regard to clients' resistance, although so far it is less explored in the field of social work research. Studies based on sequentiality are mostly strictly conversation analytical, focusing on turn-by-turn sequences of talk-in-interaction, but also include pieces of work applying membership categorisation analysis and discursive psychology (see Chapter 3). Data used in the studies are naturally occurring audio- or video-recorded interactions between professionals (doctors, therapists, counsellors, social workers etc.) and patients or clients. Studies have been conducted in different human service contexts, such as health care (Peräkylä 2002; Stivers 2005; Ijäs-Kallio *et al.* 2010), therapy (Antaki 2008; MacMartin 2008; Vehviläinen 2008; Muntigl and Choi 2010) and counselling (Vehviläinen 1999; Hutchby 2002). These settings have a lot in common with social work interaction (Jokinen *et al.* 2001; Broadhurst *et al.* 2012). Hence we discuss the results of these studies relevant to social work in the following review.

In general, resistance as sequential actions can be defined as *misalignment* or as *disaffiliation*. Alignment is used in the sense of mutual cooperation among professionals and clients, where both are orientated to similar institutional tasks and interactional agendas. Misalignment is used to mean the opposite scenario, moments of interaction in which cooperation breaks down (Zimmerman 1998: 89–90; Juhila and Abrams 2011: 286). Misalignment of clients' responses with professionals' initiations, questions and so on (resistance towards activity in progress) has especially been defined as resistance (Stivers 2005: 43; MacMartin 2008: 81–82; Hepburn and Potter 2011). Correspondingly, as Muntigl and Choi (2010: 345) write, resistance is also construed as clients' disaffiliative actions that in some ways do not conform to or support the interactional aims (or stances) of therapists or counsellors (see also Stivers 2008: 34–35). It should be noticed, however, that professionals might also produce misalignment and disaffiliation, for instance by neglecting clients' initiations and questions.

Let us now look in more detail at *how* resistant actions are accomplished in professional–client interaction according to the studies. The findings shift from *active* to *passive resistance*. The most active form is *overt resistance*, as Broadhurst *et al.* (2012: 526–528) put it: presenting direct verbal challenges to the professional's institutional and epistemological authority. For instance, the mother in child protection interaction might reject the professional's suggestion to discuss an action plan by saying 'what if your action plan is not right for me' (Broadhurst *et al.* 2012: 526). Non-affiliative responses, analysed by MacMartin (2008), are also examples of clients' overt resistance. She examined solution-focused therapy sessions and demonstrated how clients resist therapists' optimistic questions by downgrading optimism, by refocusing responses, by joking and by using sarcastic responses, as well as by complaining about optimistic questions (see also Jokinen *et al.* 2001). In its extreme form, overt resistance might mean shouting, quarrelling or walking out of meetings (Matarese and van Nijnatten under review; Caswell *et al.* 2013). Naturally, professionals can also respond with overt resistance to clients' turns, for instance by directly refusing clients' suggestions related to their services, by responding to clients' suggestions and invitations with non-sharing tones, or, sometimes, even by shouting or exiting encounters.

Offering additional or alternative information is another active form of resistance, but not as confrontational as overt resistance (Peräkylä 2002; Ijäs-Kallio *et al.* 2010: 517). For example, professionals might counter clients' troublesome self-descriptions by producing normalising talk about the mental health symptoms presented and suspected by clients as being signs of mental illnesses (Vehviläinen 1999: 134–135). When clients use this device on their part, they do not necessarily deny professional expertise or professionals' institutional authority. Instead, they provide another kind of information, often based on their own experiences, that legitimately calls into question professionals' advice, interpretations, diagnoses and so on (Peräkylä 2002; Ijäs-Kallio *et al.* 2010). Ijäs-Kallio *et al.* (2010: 511) show how the patient can challenge the doctor's diagnostic statement by providing information (such as 'how come it hurts so much?') that only the patient has access to. Clients' own experiences are often unquestioned and honoured in institutional interaction and hence are an effective means of resistance. But there are also settings in which this is not so: in psychoanalysis clients' resistance based on their own experiences can sometimes be interpreted as a sign of defensiveness and thus needs to be challenged (resisted) by the therapists (Vehviläinen 2008). In some cognitive behavioural programmes, the aim of the whole programme might be to counter (resist) the experience of being a victim and replace it with the sense of being a responsible actor.

Claims of not knowing or not remembering can also be regarded as a form of active resistance in institutional settings where talking about clients' own experiences or problems is the core of the institutional agenda. Hutchby (2002) has analysed children's 'I don't know' answers to counsellors' questions in child counselling. This kind of denial of knowledge is a powerful resistance strategy in settings where counsellors expect to elicit therapeutically relevant talk. 'I don't know' is a legitimate reason not to provide such talk and inoculates children against providing accounts. Similarly, Muntigl and Choi (2010) have noticed that 'not remembering' formulations can implement resistance to exploring deep-rooted personal or relationship problems in couple's therapy.

Possible indicators of passive resistance – used by both professionals and clients – are *unmarked acknowledgements* and *minimal responses* (e.g. 'mm', 'hm' and 'yeah') to interpretations, suggestions, advice, instructions, recommendations and so on (Heritage and Sefi 1992: 395–402; Silverman

1997: 140–145; Broadhurst *et al.* 2012: 528–530). *Total silences* might indicate the most passive form of resistant response (Raitakari 2006), and are powerful acts even though they do not include words. Silence is a very strong act of resistance, especially if it involves a refusal to take an appropriate turn. For instance, without getting any verbal responses from clients to their questions, social workers can end up with great difficulties in fulfilling their institutional tasks, such as finding out whether special child protection measures are needed.

What is then resisted in interaction by using sequential resistant actions? Clients display misalignment towards institutional tasks, interactional agendas or the aims of professionals. In more concrete terms, clients first resist professional interventions in their lives or ways of life. They implement this, for instance, by resisting professionals' advice and care plans related to their parenting and health behaviour (Heritage and Sefi 1992; Silverman 1997: 134–153; Broadhurst *et al.* 2012; Juhila *et al.* forthcoming). Second, resistance can target professional interpretations and diagnoses, such as the therapist's suggestions about the reasons for the client's mental problems (Vehviläinen 2008) or the doctor's diagnostic statements (Stivers 2005; Ijäs-Kallio *et al.* 2010). The third object of clients' resistance is the expectation to talk in a certain way when interacting. This includes resistance to therapeutically relevant talk (Hutchby 2002), such as resisting responses to optimistic questions in solution-focused therapies and social work encounters (Jokinen *et al.* 2001; MacMartin 2008) or to endeavours to improve parental engagement in child protection (Broadhurst *et al.* 2012). Lastly, resistance can focus generally on clienthood in two opposing ways. Clients can oppose their client status (such as their need for help or intervention) and the rights and responsibilities connected to it (Juhila 2003), or they can resist professionals' recommendations to terminate clienthood and to withdraw help and support (Messmer and Hitzler 2011). When it comes to the question of what professionals resist, this is a far less researched area, but, to put it simply, their resistance might target, for instance, clients' 'false' understandings of their situations, resources and problems, and clients' misaligned behaviour, as regards institutional and professional expectations.

Resistant sequential actions in interaction are non-preferred (negative) responses in the sense that they accomplish misalignment or disaffiliation to previous turns. These actions locate participants (professionals and clients) in different camps. They produce problems for the 'here and now' interaction and are therefore oriented to being something that should be discussed and solved. However, in the long run, in the forthcoming conversations among the participants, the phases of interactional resistance might be interpreted as positive forces, such as turning points in treatment processes or moments where professionals started to understand clients' points of view better.

Resistance towards stigmatised categorisations

Resistance towards stigmatised categorisations is an area of research that has been studied thoroughly in social work and related literature. The focus has been mostly on clients' self-categorisations, but resisting stigmatised client categories can also be analysed as professionals' actions. The studies are typically based on (critical) discourse analysis, on membership categorisation analysis or on narrative analysis (see Chapters 3 and 6). They most often make use of interview data (e.g. Riessman 2000; Juhila 2004; Osvaldsson 2004; Virokannas 2011), but some studies with naturally occurring institutional interaction also exist (e.g. Fox 2001; Fitzgerald and Austin 2008). Since interview data are understood and analysed as discursive and conversational talk in these studies, their findings have relevance in examining institutional social work interaction. Categories and categorisations are always inherent parts of institutional interaction (see Chapter 3) and categorisations might carry stigmas that participants in interactions make visible, for instance by resisting them. We now turn to look more closely at what is meant by resistance towards stigmatised categorisations. Where relevant, we also comment on how this resistance links to resistance as sequential actions.

Goffman's work (1961/1991 and 1964/1990) about stigmatised or spoiled identities is important here. He studied the moral careers and identities of people living in total institutions, such as prisons or mental hospitals, in a way that is very useful when studying social work settings. Life in institutions and their residents are culturally linked with negative characteristics; people who have ended up there are thought to have failed in their lives in one way or another. This is how stigmatised categories of places and their residents emerge. In his essays on stigma, Goffman underlines that persons as such are not to be understood as stigmatised, but stigma is always generated in social situations, in interactions between people in certain contexts (Slembrouck and Hall 2003: 45). Hence, the focus of research should be on interactional categorisation processes.

The categorisation of people always has two aspects. On the one hand, it preserves harmony in society and facilitates orientation to and encounters with people in different situations. On the other hand, categorisation can just as easily maintain discrimination in producing 'identity prisons' charged with negative characteristics for some people (Silverman 1998: 88). Those assigned to the negative, stigmatising categories cannot ignore them. When people refer to themselves in different contexts, they tend to comply with the expectations of other people. In other words, they use identities that others can recognise (Gubrium and Holstein 2001: 7). Matters become complicated if co-participants expect and offer a stigmatised categorisation membership to a person, which is often the case in social work interaction. It is understandably difficult to accept such identity categorisations totally, without any acts of resistance (Juhila 2004).

What categorisations do social work clients then recognise as stigmatised and needing resistance? Those that define them as deficient, incapable, deviant or troublesome, such as those of homeless or unemployed persons, inadequate parents, substance abusers, or problematically behaving and delinquent young people (Juhila and Abrams 2011: 286–287). Studies show *how* people resist these kinds of negative and stereotyping categories being associated with them in several ways. In social work interactions resistance can be realised in and through sequential actions, using both active and passive forms of resistance. But there are also special devices related to resisting stigmas.

An important resisting strategy towards stigmatised categorisations is what Sacks (1963/1984) calls '*on doing being ordinary*'. When using this strategy, clients' talk counters the stigma ascribed to them by presenting themselves as normal and displaying normal interaction, thereby downgrading problem categories (van Nijnatten 2013). For instance, Osvaldsson (2004) shows how female residents in youth detention homes specialising in assessments and/or treatment use the notions of normality when describing their presumably deviant behaviour. They do this typically by relocating the notion of deviance from the subject herself to the social circumstances. Similarly, Juhila (2004) demonstrates how homeless persons living in a shelter stress the ordinary quality of the shelter and its residents (this is the place where quite ordinary, although unlucky, citizens live) or their own ordinariness (although I live here, I am an ordinary person). In social work interaction the strategy of doing ordinariness or normality might be in use by professionals too. They can, for example, diminish clients' problem talk by emphasising the normality of the described matter (e.g. 'sometimes we all have concerns of not fulfilling the criteria of good motherhood').

Another way to resist categories is to describe oneself with *competing categories* that makes the membership of stigmatised categories questionable or irrelevant. For instance, persons who have been defined as long-term unemployed can present themselves as permanently sick persons and thus eligible for a pension and membership in the category group of retirees (Caswell *et al.* 2011; Välimaa 2011). Professionals can also use stigma-reducing categories, such as by referring to more empowering categories instead of problem-based client categories when describing and evaluating clients' situations.

Resistance toward stigmatised categorisations in its extreme mode can be termed *fighting back*, meaning a total *rejection* of the ascribed spoiled identities. In the course of social work interaction, rejection is done with active and overt turns of resistance. Virokannas (2011: 338–340) uses the concept of fighting back in her analysis of the categorisation of motherhood in the context of drug abuse and child welfare services. She shows how the client, who sees her identity as a mother being totally and wrongly undermined by the social worker, demands that this categorisation should be retracted. Simultaneously, she rejects the category membership of a child welfare client. In practice, social work settings are sometimes based on involuntary clienthood. This means that 'just walking out' and rejecting one's category as a client is not possible, or has at least serious sanctions and consequences for the person in question. So far there seems to be very little research evidence of this kind of 'walking out' resistance occurring in social work interaction. Correspondingly, there is a lack of research on 'not walking in' or not selecting clienthood in more voluntarily based social work settings, which could be interpreted as resistance towards the anticipated stigma associated with clienthood.

Resistance towards clients' stigmatised categorisations can be shared actions by professionals and clients and thus be oriented as a positive force in social work interaction. Through resistance these two parties might construct themselves as allies in fighting against cultural stigmas. However, another option is that resistance divides them into different camps, especially in such institutional interactions where professionals persuade or insist that clients accept such categories, which clients resist as spoiled and stigmatised.

Resistance towards institutional and governmental policies

Resisting stigmatised identities, as discussed above, relates to negative characteristics linked culturally to certain categorisations of people. We now move on from cultural issues to policy-level issues dealing with resistance towards institutional and governmental policies, although these two dimensions of resistance are often connected to each other. The policy-level line of research draws commonly on critical discourse analysis founded on Foucault's (1981) work on power, knowledge and resistance, and on his followers' writings about the analytics of government (Dean 1999; Rose 2002). The studies often have an ethnographic orientation and use multiple ways of gathering data (observations, documents, interviews), including naturally occurring social work interaction. Unlike studies about stigma, this research focuses more on professionals' than on clients' resistance. Resistance towards institutional and governmental policies fits well with what Thomas and Davies (2005: 683) call the *micro-politics of resistance*. They strive to break the dualistic debate of 'compliance with' versus 'resistance to'. Professionals and clients cannot totally ignore or reject institutional and governmental policies, but they can resist them with multiple subtle means, and sometimes in more overt ways, in everyday institutional interaction. We see the micro-politics of resistance as something that can be accomplished in social work interaction. Similarly, as is the case in resisting stigmatised categorisations, this resistance can be displayed in interaction by using sequential resistant actions.

What institutional and governmental policies have then been perceived as targets of the professionals' micro-politics of resistance? To summarise, the targets of resistance are various governmental or institutional policy changes. In other words, they are new policies that are implemented, and to which professionals and clients must respond. The most studied area of the micro-politics of resistance has been different managerial endeavours that are seen to limit professionals' discretion and hinder client-led work, and therefore calls for resistance (Hjörne *et al.* 2010). For instance, researchers have demonstrated that professionals resist managerial reforms in psychiatric care (Saario 2012), performance management models that are implemented through new information technologies in child care (Wastell *et al.* 2010; White *et al.* 2010), 'punitive managerialism', which is the managerial mode of practice and the control of risky populations in probation practice (Gregory 2010), and the demands of economic effectiveness in the context of supported housing (Saario and Raitakari 2010).

Clients can obviously also resist policy changes and managerial endeavours. Caswell *et al.* (2013) have analysed clients' responses to the activation policy in the context of active employment policy in job centres. Some of the clients openly resist the activation demands and the positive narrative framework related to it. Since the goals of creating active, participating and responsible clients are emphasised in many organisations and in governmental policy papers, similar demands are present, and possibly resisted, in other social work settings (e.g. Eskelinen *et al.* 2010; Solberg 2011; Wilinska and Henning 2011; Caswell *et al.* 2013). For example, Broadhurst *et al.* (2012) examine how the goal of engaging parents in child protection practice is not always shared by the clients and is sometimes even confronted.

How do professionals and clients resist policies in institutional interaction? Professionals often use *subtle strategies* that do not totally reject suggested policy changes. This resonates well with Foucault's (1981: 95) understanding of resistance: 'where there is power, there is resistance, and yet, or rather consequently, this resistance is never in a position of exteriority in relation to power'. As Saario (2012: 1) states: 'instead of strongly challenging managerial reforms, practitioners keep them alive and ongoing by continuously improvising, criticizing and dismissing reforms' non-functional features'. Using humour to challenge instructions coming from above can also be one form of subtle resistance (Griffiths 1998). So, focusing on everyday encounters, resistance towards institutional and governmental policies can be observed as less of a dismissive and oppositional activity, and more in terms of being 'routinized, informal and inconspicuous' (Thomas and Davies 2005: 686). In the course of institutional interaction this means the use of less active and less overt actions of resistance. Similar forms of subtle resistance might be present when analysing clients' ways of using the micro-politics of resistance. For instance, Solberg (2011) has noticed that, although the clients in activation encounters do not have the explicit plans for their future that are demanded of them, they manage to give relevant accounts for not having them. So they do not totally reject the expectation to make a plan, but resist it by explaining why making it is not now possible or reasonable for them (cf. offering additional information as resistance).

In the previous section we addressed the lack of research on clients' 'walking out' or 'not walking in' resistance. When it comes to resisting institutional or governmental policies some research can be found. A recent Danish study of the use of economic sanctions towards cash benefit recipients shows how these clients sometimes walk out of the welfare system for a period of time as a consequence of the sanctions (Caswell et al. 2011). Research on homeless people living on the street (bag-people) has shown that some of these very marginalised people resist the demands of the system, not necessarily as a reflected, deliberate choice, but nevertheless as resistance towards demands in terms of being registered, talking to professionals, having to enter offices and so on (Caswell and Schultz 2001). This resistance tends to be in the shape of 'not walking in'.

In spite of the fact that there seems to be little research on *overt resistance* towards polices, the possible existence and relevance of this should not be dismissed. However, as more than an empirical issue accomplished in institutional practices, this topic has been approached as a 'should be' issue. For instance, Carey (2008) argues that professionals' resistance towards prevailing ideologies (e.g. neoliberalism and new public management) tends to be individualistic, dispersed and sporadic, and thus there is a need for greater exposure to 'emancipatory' ideologies, for instance in professional education.

As was the case with actions resisting stigmas, resistance towards institutional and governmental policies can unite professionals and clients as allies (with common enemies) or as being in different camps (one persuading and demanding that the other accepts and follows policies, the other resisting them).

Resistance in social work interaction: data examples and analyses

We will now proceed to analyse the concept of resistance through the use of naturally occurring interaction in social work. The empirical data will illustrate a wide variety of the 'whats' and 'hows' of resistance displayed in the previous part of this chapter. It should be noticed, however, that the most extreme and also rare forms of resistance, such as shouting, overt quarrelling and walking out, are not present in the data. The data are located in two different institutional contexts: social work with sick benefit recipients in a Danish job centre and mental health and substance abuse work in a Finnish supported housing unit targeted at service users suffering from both mental health and substance abuse problems.

A professional–client meeting in a job centre

The first empirical example stems from a meeting between a social worker (SW) and a client (C) in a Danish job centre. The institutional task of the centre is to activate clients who are unemployed or are otherwise outside the labour market, but also to assess their ability to work. The client, Peter, is a sick benefit recipient, who has a long history of clienthood in the centre. He is around 50 years old and has a wife and two children. He has serious back pains and has recently had an operation. He uses a lot of medication to handle his pain and is visibly uncomfortable during the interaction. He has previously worked as a truck driver and talks about having a strong labour market identity. The interaction of the meeting between the social worker and the client is, overall, positive and constructive. The participants have met each other several times in the centre before this meeting.

Extract 1

```
1    SW:   but Peter what I have to (.) if I shall help you through this
2          legislation because we will be: faced with (.) that it is probably
3          (.) that we have to think about (.) maybe some other forms of welfare
4          support than sick benefit
5    C:    °yes°
6    SW:   then I need some documentation (.) I simply have to have your
7          ability to work (.) described (.) described more thoroughly
8          than what we have now (1) what you can do [and
9    C:                                              [°yes°
10   SW:   and what it is [that
11   C:                   [yeah
12   SW:   and I have some suggestions I just want to talk to you about
13         what I can see as possibilities right now that I can try to include (.)
14         these are not in a work place but will enable assessment nonetheless
15         (1) but one way to put it (2) I have the option that I can (.) send
16         an occupational therapist to your home to follow you for a whole
17         day and describe your functioning level I know you have already
18         told me this but to have a professional person documenting this (.)
19         then you can say (.) then maybe she will (.) follow you for half
20         of the day (.) in the morning in your home and say what is (.)
21         what is your functioning level (1) you can say (.) that is an option (1)
22         another option [is
23   C:                   [no that is too bloody embarrassing
24         ((laughs a bit)) no I simply won't (.) [no
25   SW:                                          [you can't think like that Peter
26   C:    no ((laughs a bit)) no but honestly (1)
27   SW:   another option could be ((goes on to explain possible
28         activation/rehabilitation measures))
```

The client, Peter, resists the attempt by the social worker to have his functional level evaluated. His resistance is directed towards being a client, who is continuously evaluated in relation to his (lack of) ability to work. This is a central issue of clienthood when it comes to clients in job centres. First, he resists by using minimal acknowledgements, speaking with a low tone of voice and only using monosyllabic responses (lines 5, 9 and 11). At the end of the extract he uses overt resistance, saying straight out that he simply will not accept the option proposed by the social worker of having an occupational therapist visit his home in order to describe his functional level: it is too embarrassing (lines 23–24 and 26). He does not only resist the idea of having his functioning level described (although the interaction indicates that both the social worker and the client find that the demand for further documentation is a strong institutional demand), but he also resists the idea of having someone come to the intimacy of his home in order to describe his functioning level. He uses a swear word to underline his resistance ('bloody'). The emphasis of the word 'embarrassing' and laughing are also signs of resistance. He does not get angry with the social worker, but rather appeals to her understanding by saying 'honestly'. She responds to this by coming up with an alternative option.

The client uses resistance in the interaction, but resistance can also be seen on the part of the social worker. Her use of resistance is very subtle, but it is directed towards the institutional procedures she is expected to follow and to demand the client follow too. In her long turn in the middle of the extract (lines 12–22) she uses pauses and restarts sentences often, showing her resistance towards the message she is trying to get across to Peter, namely that he needs to have his lack of ability to work described and documented in order to move the case forward. Furthermore, the extract shows how resistance is also something that is used actively in the interaction, as the social worker addresses the anticipated resistance from the client ('I know you have already told me this, but', lines 17–18).

Further on in the meeting the conversation addresses the length of time needed in order to gain sufficient documentation to proceed with the possible application for early retirement/a disability pension. We will look closer at the resistance involved in this below.

Extract 2

```
1  SW:   and well (.) I am thinking a bit along the lines of (.) of course
2        you have to have until the end of May to finish your
3        [rehabilitation training and at present we are in late April
4  C:    [yes
5  SW:   what I would like is that when the rehabilitation training
6        ((physical training at the hospital)) ends (.) we will (1) then
```

7		[we will do (.) the occupational (3) assessment
8	C:	[yes
9	SW:	at the same time as we gather the medical documentation
10		because there is no point in protracting it
11	C:	no
12	SW:	we might as well say that while we do the assessment we
13		will get the papers concerning health issues so that we have
14		medical statements and an occupational assessment from
15		the ((name of activation offer)) (.)
16	C:	but well yes [yes I see your problem (.)
17	SW:	[yes
18	C:	but really (6) we can't avoid it being protracted
19	SW:	yes that is really what we should do Peter
20	C:	I see (.)
21	SW:	when you think protracted what is on your mind
22	C:	it is because (.) because (.) I think (.) I think (.) well I think
23		that it is a bottomless pit always (.) it is as if it has been
24		going on for a long time now so (.) in one way or another
25		one sort of (.) one sort of has come to the point now where
26		one (.) would really like some peace and quiet (.)
27	SW:	yes
28	C:	I feel as if one keeps being chased around you know (.)

In this extract we see resistance also directed at demands that stem from institutional and governmental policy level. The social worker addresses the need for specific types of documentation (lines 12–15) and the client responds to this by placing the need for documentation on the social worker as part of the institutional set-up by saying 'I see your problem' (line 16). However, they continue straight on to addressing the danger of the process being protracted, which they both resist. The social worker's resistance is focused on getting the necessary documentation quickly and with the right timing in order to avoid protraction. The resistance of the client – which can even be characterised as fighting back – is directed at the very concept of clienthood, which he talks about as never-ending ('a bottomless pit', 'has been going on for a long time now', lines 23–24) and as something that includes being chased around – a stigmatised category he does not wish to continue being placed within. Peter displays hesitance (and resistance) in his responses starting with 'but' (line 16) and including a long pause (line 18) regarding whether they can really avoid protraction and the 'bottomless' clienthood with the strategy offered by the social worker (lines 12–15).

At the same time, however, Peter also resists the idea of being 'a pensioner', which is addressed in the following extract from the last part of the interaction.

Extract 3

```
1   C:      yes (1) well (.) every now and then (1) we have talked about
2           this at home (.) every now and then (.) you know (.) living
3           the life of a pensioner is just not worthy because (2) when
4           you don't feel well what should you do with your time (.)
5           other than feel poorly
6   SW:     °no° (.) Peter you have to try to understand it is also
7           important for your family that maybe also that you can have
8           some peace and quiet regarding the financial [side of things
9   C:                                                   [yes yes there is of
10          course that [yes
11  SW:                 [and even if one becomes a pensioner Peter then it
12          is not the same as saying that one cannot have a job of some
13          sort (.) one is allowed to earn a certain amount even if
14          one is on an early retirement pension
```

The client resists the category of 'a pensioner' (someone who receives early retirement/a disability pension), as he defines it as a life without value, an unworthy life (lines 2–5). He resists this category, while simultaneously working on 'doing being ordinary' (Sacks 1963/1984) – being someone who can still participate in the labour market (competing categories). However, while resisting the category of a pensioner he also agrees with the positive aspects of 'peace and quiet' anticipated by the social worker (line 8), which are essentially part of the very same category within the active labour market policy framework. The social worker addresses his resistance by attempting to redefine the very category of a pensioner. Rather than being a category for those with an unworthy life, she highlights the category as being one in which the financial situation is clear and one that does not exclude participation in the labour market of some sort (lines 11–14). Thus she works at building a bridge between the category resisted by Peter and those addressed positively by the client throughout the interaction.

A case conference in a supported housing unit

We now turn to our second empirical example, which comes from a case conference held in a Finnish supported housing unit targeted for service users suffering from both mental health and substance abuse problems. The objective of the case conference is to assess how the client is coping with her housing and with her methadone treatment. The participants at the case conference are the client, Erica, two professionals from the supported housing unit (who don't talk in the extract) and two municipal commissioners – one who is responsible for coordinating special housing services and another who is responsible for coordinating methadone treatment.

Erica is a woman under 30 who has used drugs for several years. Due to her substance abuse she also occasionally suffers from psychotic and physical symptoms.

Erica talks in a quiet voice and rather little at the conference, but still she takes and is also given a strong position to state her perceptions and opinions. This does not mean, however, that the professionals are not the ones setting the agenda of the conference, leading the talk and having the ultimate power to make decisions concerning Erica's housing and treatment. The conference interaction is similar to an interview format (Silverman 1997), where the professionals (mostly the methadone treatment coordinator) pose the questions and Erica is expected to provide answers. In the course of the conference both professionals and Erica resist each other's stances and views in a subtle manner – so that the conference may continue without an overt dispute. This can be seen through a cautious and delicate way of talking and interacting (see Chapter 9). In the following extract the methadone treatment coordinator (P1), the commissioner (P2) and Erica (C) discuss Erica's drug use and the proper dose of methadone in her treatment. Erica resists a suggestion to lower the amount of medication. In methadone treatment clients are expected to follow strict treatment plans, to be willing to gradually lower the amount of medication and not to use other drugs during treatment. The professionals are talking these institutional policy level expectations into being while Erica shows some resistance towards them. The extract also demonstrates what tricky and delicate issues drug use and methadone treatment are both culturally and morally.

Extract 4

1	P1:	were you then when we last met (.) about that time
2		using lyrica or benzos
3	C:	no (2) that (.) merely methadone (.) it makes me like (.)
4		sleepy and (2) I often start to nod off in afternoon (.) even
5		though the dose is so small 65 so still
6	P1:	when was it last assessed [your dosage (.)
7	C:	[well
8	P1:	if you describe symptoms like that
9	C:	(6) erm (6)
10	P1:	when have you remembered to talk about it to doctor
11	C:	I haven't talked about it since (2) it doesn't bother me that condition
12	P2:	would it be worthwhile now when you go to hospital to talk about it
13		to ((name of the doctor))
14	C:	so I need to observe if I still have that (2) that wooziness
15	P1:	because yes it also (.) also then it disrupts [how much you are able to
16	C:	[°hmm°
17	P1:	participate in activities or to do things you wished to do here

```
18              ((at the supported housing unit)) or [elsewhere (.) that about
19   C:                                            [yes
20   P1:    and then of course the doctor will tell you honestly if she does not
21          want to lower that dose for the reason (.) that it takes it to risk limits
22          (.) that it exposes you to getting more drugs by yourself
23   C:     °yes°
24   P1:    those (medicine) changes are done very slowly (.) but yes usually
25          then after certain time they start to drop off little by little the [°dose° (.)
26   C:                                                                         [°hmm°
27   P1:    but of course not so that (.) that (.) [you should have to go and replace it
28   C:                                            [°hmm°
29   P1:    with some other drug this thought may be there in the background (.) they
30          haven't yet started to discuss (.) the dose with you
31   C:     hmm
32   P2:    how about (.) ((the name of supported housing unit)) supervisors' (.)
33          point of view on this (.) now that Erica has been here for a month
34          how has Erica managed and acted here (2) in the community
35          and (.) has she been able to join the group
```

The first professional (P1) starts the sequence with a straight question (lines 1–2), which includes a suspicion and indirect accusation that the client had used other drugs during the treatment period. Erica overtly resists the suspicion (and thus the professional's interpretation) by saying no and offering additional information and an alternative explanation for her condition in the previous meeting (lines 3–5). Her experience is that the small dose of methadone makes her sleepy, not sedatives. The professional assesses the condition the client has just described as undesirable and suspects that the size of the present dose is not right. This can be read through her question and remark ('when was it last assessed your dosage (.) if you describe symptoms like that', lines 6 and 8). The client resists the prospect embedded in the question (that the dose should perhaps be lowered) in a subtle manner by a minimal response (line 7) and an extraordinarily long total silence (line 9).

The professional responds to Erica's passive resistance by posing a follow-up question that still indicates that the dosage should be checked (line 10). The client's answer and way of talking include resistance; she gives an answer that reveals that she has not been active in bringing up the need to lower the dose (line 11). Thus her responses are not in line with the expectations related to a 'proper' client identity in a methadone treatment programme. Erica justifies 'not talking' to the doctor by appealing to her experience and will; for her the current condition is not a problem. Next, another professional (P2) takes a turn and resists the client's justification by also suggesting a discussion with the doctor (lines 12–13). Thus alignment between the two professionals is created.

The last suggestion is given in the form of personalised advice (see Chapter 7), the function of which might be to soften professional intervention. The advice turn shows that the professional takes into account the client's resistant stance and tries to persuade the client to reconsider her opinion. But the turn is not successful in persuading her. Instead of reconsidering her opinion, Erica continues resisting by offering additional information. This time she does it by undermining her own previous assessment that methadone would make her sleepy (line 14). Maybe the reported symptom has disappeared and, if it has, there is no need to make any changes to the amount of dose.

The professionals bypass the client's additional information – they resist it passively – and instead Professional 1 starts to talk about the downside of the wooziness (lines 15, 17–18). The resistance is challenged by reminding the client that she herself had previously wished to be able to participate more in activities. As a response to the client's resistance, Professional 1 also provides further information about methadone treatment, by ensuring that the reduction of the dose is done little by little and not in such a way that she would be pushed to relapse (lines 20–22, 24–25, 27 and 29–30). Erica responds to this talk with minimal responses (lines 23, 26, 28 and 31). She does not overtly reject the assumption that she would be at risk of being driven to the simultaneous use of other drugs. However, subtle resistance and discomfort with the topic, the client category on offer and the expectations related to it seem to still be present in the client's talk. Her responses are minimal and she does not disclose or elaborate her thoughts in such a manner as might be expected from a 'good' methadone treatment client (Juhila 2003). After the client's last minimal response, Professional 2 changes the addressee of the talk (and the topic) and asks from the professionals working in the supported housing unit how the client has coped there.

Implications for social work practice

In this chapter we have demonstrated that resistance has multiple targets, forms and functions ('whats' and 'hows') in everyday social work practices. Resistance is common and constantly present but not always easily recognisable in social work practice. We suggest that it deserves careful attention when developing social work as human interaction work and research. Resistance comprises many meanings and messages – there is always a reason for resistance.

In professional social work discourse, resistance is commonly seen as being the clients' fixed, problematic attitude and behaviour. In this chapter we have argued for the importance of understanding how confrontation based on clients' resistance is present, produced and dealt with in naturally occurring social work interaction. The focus then is not on resistant clients as a readymade category but on the processes where certain categories, as well as resistance, are talked into being. Resistance and client categorisation are accomplished in actions, and it becomes a possible resource in a particular interactional setting. For instance, in our example in which Erica's situation is discussed, the client can be seen to be categorised both as non-adherent and 'non-behaving' (not agreeing with or following the idea of the treatment programme) as well as a strong actor (presenting her own assessments and experienced needs) due to her resistance.

Interactional analysis also reveals that both clients and professionals display resistance, and this is done *in situ* during interaction. In Erica's case the professional does not approve of the client's point of view but resists it by giving new information and persuading her to follow the treatment programme and agree to lower the amount of medication. This self-evident and simple finding is important, since it calls into question some presumed premises of the social work profession. Social work is based on certain normative expectations of a good life and how it can be reached. If clients seem to disagree with these expectations, they are easily categorised as being on the wrong track. When professionals 'guide' clients back to the right track in these kinds of situations, it is not usually understood as resistance towards clients' ways of life but just as a morally correct way to act.

Seeing resistance through the lens of confrontation between clients and professionals is not the only way that professional discourse makes sense of resistance. Understanding these two parties as possible allies is another option. The flavour of this kind of joint resistance can be identified in our first example, in which Peter resists frustrated documentation demands in a job centre and the social worker displays understanding towards such resistance. Although the social worker argues that they have to follow the institutional rules and procedures, she still does not defend them strongly, but rather implies that she regards them as frustrating as well. Joint resistance can be easily targeted at these kinds of institutional and governmental policies but also at culturally stigmatised categorisations. As Peter's case demonstrates, joint resistance is commonly produced in subtle ways during the course of interaction, and thus only a detailed study of social worker–client encounters makes it visible. There is a risk that we miss and bypass the possibilities that subtle resistance sequences have in strengthening client–professional relations and in questioning existing procedures, policies and power structures.

As we mentioned above, professional social work discourse usually associates resistance with clients' identities or actions. The same emphasis is found in research on client–professional interaction. Similar to this, our two examples and their analyses start from the clients' resistant acts. 'A resistance sequence' is commonly seen to proceed like this: the professional makes a suggestion/interpretation/intervention, gives advice etc. → the client resists → the professional responds to the resistance (often by resisting it).

However, this emphasis alone is not enough, since it *'hides' professionals' resistant actions and clients' suggestions*. The resistance sequence can also proceed in the opposite direction: the client makes a suggestion/interpretation/intervention, gives advice etc. → the professional resists → the client responds to the resistance. For instance, Erica's case could be read from this 'other way around': she suggests that there is no need to talk with the doctor about the dosage but the professional resists the suggestion, which is followed by Erica's response, defending her suggestions. This kind of 'other way around' analysis (concentrating on the professionals' resistant actions) is important, especially from the point of view of client participation/involvement/centredness as emphasised strongly in professional social work discourse (see Matarese and van Nijnatten under review).

Resistance in social work interaction is bound to the moral and ethical issues unavoidable in any social work practice. It is a matter of local negotiation, whether resistance is assessed as morally right or wrong, or as a positive or negative force. Is resistance seen as justified (and for whom?) towards certain managerial endeavours, towards administrative documentation demands or towards expectations to follow the plans of treatment/recovery programmes? How about resistance towards accepting one's guilt or responsibilities in violent or criminal behaviour, or towards helping a client in need? When is it right to attempt to break down resistance, and when is the other person's resistance interpreted as feedback, leading one to correct one's actions and behaviour?

To sum up, resistance is neither just bad/good or a problem/resource in social work interaction but can be both, depending on how it is produced, discussed and negotiated in local practices. It is thus not possible to create general guidelines on how to deal with clients' or professionals' resistance in interaction, but instead we wish to emphasise the importance of recognising the multiple targets, forms and functions of resistance in social work practices. Resistance is meaningful and should be treated as important information in social work interaction. Resistance tells us what accounts the clients and the professionals are ready/able to accept and see as reasonable and morally justified in particular situations. By having an open and analytic view on resistance we learn important things about professional culture and the clients' ways of defining and understanding their own situations.

9

DELICACY

Carolus van Nijnatten and Eero Suoninen

Social work belongs to the social midfield that mediates between individual and society. Social workers deal with citizens who, for all kinds of reasons, are threatened with losing their grip on their lives. Since autonomy is a core value in western societies, issues in this field may easily be considered delicate. This may refer to questions that have a direct effect on economic or physical independence, but also to questions that have an indirect relation to autonomy, for example the anxiety of becoming isolated because of one's different nature or background (e.g. homosexuality, ethnic minority, intellectual disability). Having serious problems in one's life already may be confusing because one cannot continue one's role performance (Gross and Stone 1964) and needs professional help. Most of the interaction between social workers and their clients refers to this type of problem. That makes social work communication a complex and tense co-construction of shared understanding rather than a means of simply transmitting and receiving messages. Maintenance of independence is such a crucial issue for most people that the very appearance of a social worker, which may be an indication that independence is no longer granted, may already arouse hostile responses. Anticipating such sensitivity, social workers try to wriggle out of confrontation by careful formulations. Consider the following example of a social worker's (family supervisor – FS) talk to a mother:

> FS: [. . .] yes quite once in a while something might be said like yes listen here uh [pause] for Jacqueline it would uh perhaps also uh this or not perhaps but that would be <u>better</u> for her upbringing and it could perhaps happen quite once in a while and again it remains (.) open (.) I'll also ask you openly about it.

In this fragment (van Nijnatten *et al.* 2001) the family supervisor tries to explain the changes in parental authority as a consequence of a family supervision order. Her wordings are unspecific and indirect. The use of interjections such as 'might', 'would' and 'could perhaps' are efforts to mitigate the impact of the family intervention for the parents. The supervisor's formal authority is hinted at by unspecific formulations such as 'something', 'it', 'that', 'it remains open'. By using the passive voice she tries to distract the attention from her capacity to intervene at the cost of parental power.

In this chapter, we will focus on the issue of marking topics as delicate, which we call 'doing delicacy'. Social workers and their clients often find themselves in communicative situations that may become sensitive, embarrassing and upsetting. We will pay attention to the subtlety of the means that social workers and their clients have at their disposal when creating shared understanding about potentially delicate issues.

First, we will present the theoretical origins of the idea of studying doing delicacy in human services interaction and review the essential research on the subject. From this review we collect the tools for the analysis of social work interactions. We will then present two illustrations of how these tools may be used. The first illustration originates from probation work, the second one from child welfare work. Finally, we return to the question of what is the relevance of doing delicacy in social work interactions.

Theoretical origins of the idea of studying delicacy

There are two traditional ways to explain people's behaviour when sensitivity is at stake. One view emphasises individual cognitions. Personal understanding is considered a reason for a certain message to become delicate: the relevance for the life of the receiver of the message (e.g. the outcome of a job interview), the way that person usually deals with problematic issues (e.g. self-control), and the extent to which the problematic content of the message is seen as something inescapable (e.g. an incurable disease). In the other traditional perspective conventions representing cultural rules and values determine the social value of certain issues, and how one should deal with them in public and private environments.

In symbolic interactionist theories, these explanations of sensitivity are put into a more complicated perspective, as it is suggested that people, in their daily actions, take other people's views into consideration. The most famous representative of this school, Mead (1935), suggested that it is important for a human to take other people's attitudes into account. 'The other' and 'the generalised other' are conditional for the way people think and interact within society. This perspective that emphasises interaction in spite of personal features or cultural rules was developed further by Goffman (1959), who presents social interaction as a dramaturgical performance, in which people try to manage the impressions they make and are busy preserving social relations by preventing loss of face for others and themselves. Since Goffman's publications (1959, 1961/1991, 1974), many linguistically oriented social scientists have continued this line of reasoning, suggesting that human understanding and activities are jointly created and re-created, in and through ongoing negotiations by the participants of interaction. This reasoning can be found in traditions of ethnomethodology (e.g. Garfinkel 1967; Sacks 1992), social constructionism (e.g. Shotter 1993; Gergen 1994), conversation analysis (e.g. Drew and Heritage 1992b; Silverman 1997) and discourse analysis (e.g. Potter and Wetherell 1987; Potter 1996).

Accepting the idea that people's behaviour can only be adequately understood in interactions with other people, we conclude that neither individual cognitions nor cultural rules can entirely explain what people do in interactions. Concerning the theme of this chapter this means, as many social scientists maintain (e.g. Heath 1988; Maynard 1991; Bergmann 1992; Silverman 1997), that the sensitivity of uttering issues depends more on social reflecting and interactional dynamics than on the unidirectional effects of culture or cognition.

To study delicacy as an interactional phenomenon we need to analyse the details of interaction in real everyday situations. The first task then is to identify which issues in the interactions are *marked* as delicate rather than deciding beforehand which ones are usually sensitive. This kind of marking may include both categorisations and sequential features present in conversation. Some categories or themes may be indicated beforehand as 'hot topics' – for example sexuality, death and cruelty – but it is only by its presentation and treatment in the actual conversation that one can see whether an issue actually becomes delicate and how the marking of delicacy is done. In addition, sensitivity is a co-construction, which means that it becomes relevant to analyse this phenomenon as a co-creative process of accepting, avoiding, opposing and mystifying. We use the term 'doing delicacy' to indicate various kinds of interactional strategies that are relevant in this constructive process: indirectness of expression, expressive caution and any kind of deviation from straightforward, immediate, explicit and unambiguous expression or implications of things and issues.

There are two relevant and partly overlapping theoretical perspectives on the analysis of doing delicacy: one that focuses on details of expressive caution in the course of interaction (Bergmann 1992; Silverman 1997) and another that focuses on morality of categories that are referred to or hinted at in conversation (Silverman 1997). The study of *expressive caution* is based on the idea that words may be interpreted in multiple ways (e.g. Goffman 1955, 1959; Garfinkel 1967). In intercultural communication, there are many examples of situations that are interpreted as 'face-threatening' (Goffman 1955) by one of the participants while being judged positively by another participant. One strategy to address this problem of ambiguity is to 'mark' (or index) words by using different tones or by adding explanations. The analysis of expressive caution is relevant in contexts in which speakers display sensitivity towards potentially embarrassing matters.

The *morality of categories* is related to the work of Sacks (1972a, 1992) on the 'membership categorisation device' (MCD) and scholars of 'membership categorisation analysis' (MCA). Categories may be identified and oriented to by the means of 'category-bound activities' (CBAs) or other category-bound features. Hence regularly used categories may be identified by analysing participants' references, hints or associations to these categories. Silverman (1987: 233–265) has developed the idea that, in addition to general categories and category devices employed usually in MCA (e.g. standard relational pairs such as child/mother), it is possible to analyse how more specified categories (e.g. autonomous child/non-interventionist mother *or* aggrieved daughter/neurotic mother) are used. By such data-driven explication it is possible to analyse subtle balancing between possible identity-constructions in the course of interaction (Silverman 1987: 237). The most common example in the context of social work is that balancing between institutional (social) requirements and individual interests of citizens is essential (Hjörne *et al.* 2010). This kind of balancing, which is often done by mentioning category-bound features that refer or hint to certain categories, brings moral dimensions into interaction. If we try to understand how people negotiate what is suitable and morally acceptable and legitimate activity, it is relevant to study both when and how people mark topics as delicate and when they hint at certain categories.

Studies on delicacy in social services' interaction

The theme of doing delicacy is not common in social work studies. Most influential publications were written in the 1990s in the field of health studies. Recently there have been connections in the field of social work research to these studies both as a main topic and also as an additional topic of different kinds of studies focused on social work interaction. Four key publications from the 1990s are worth mentioning here:

- Maynard (1991) explains the perspective-display series in which one participant tries to understand the other's perception of a delicate issue by taking the other's expression of his or her perspective as a starting point for expressing his/her own perspective. Such a strategy enables a professional to announce bad news or otherwise confronting information in such a way that the client's perspective has been taken into account.
- Bergmann (1992) analysed psychiatric intake interviews and found many forms of expressive caution, foreshadowing potentially delicate

matters. He noticed that psychiatrists proceeded by proffering informa- tion or impressions rather than asking interrogative questions. This is recurrently done by the use of 'litotes', which are assertions that deny the opposite of what is being indicated. The use of litotes relieves the speaker of the task of specifying what one is talking about and invites the interviewee to identify an unspecified issue. Softening words may function as caution and discretion and mark upcoming potentially delicate issues.

- Linell and Bredmar (1996) analysed how potentially delicate topics were dealt with in interactions between newly pregnant women and midwives in a primary health care unit. Linell and Bredmar identified typical patterns of indirectness and mitigation that may point to a strategy to deal with delicacy. Indirectness and mitigation were analysed in relation to midwives' questions about (1) smoking and drinking, (2) HIV and syphilis and (3) malformation and possible abortion. Smoking and drinking were dealt with in an immediate way, by the use of softening words and a limited depth of penetration. By contrast, HIV and syphilis were introduced through reframing and a delayed approach.

- Silverman (1997) analysed interactions between HIV counsellors and clients. He found that counsellors and patients use expressive caution (delay of delivery, various speech perturbations) and elaborations and story prefaces to mark potentially delicate objects. Counsellors also use many devices (e.g. perspective display sequences, downgrades, indirect questions and justifications) to provide a favourable environment for disclosing delicate information, starting with unproblematic questions and compliments to put patients in a positive light. Patients produce a minimal amount of potentially delicate items. Like counsellors, patients prefer to start with unproblematic information. Silverman suggests, leaning on the detailed analysis of participants' interactional cues, that the core of empathic counselling interaction is not the interplay of two private selves, but rather the interplay of actions making use of publicly available apparatuses of description ('categorisation devices').

All of these scholars studied delicacy as a phenomenon that is constructed in and through the interaction of institutional communication. They based their studies on analysis of transcriptions of conversations between professionals and clients. Other publications (Sacks 1972a; Heath 1988; Silverman and Peräkylä 1990; Maynard 1991; Weijts et al. 1993) relate to the four texts described above and also underline that delicacy is the result of interactional cooperation of the conversation partners marking sensitive issues rather than attributing cultural dominant values or individual psychological states of mind.

In social work research there are several studies that continue this line of analytical work (Suoninen 1999; van Nijnatten 2005 and forthcoming;

Noordegraaf *et al.* 2009). In addition, many researchers who are interested in advice-giving (Silverman 1997: 109–182), persuasion (Suoninen and Jokinen 2005) and interactional positions (Suoninen and Wahlström 2009) have taken doing delicacy as one aspect of their thematically focused analysis.

Formulation

In the literature discussed above we found several conversational strategies aimed at inciting disclosure by comforting the conversation. These studies focus on the relevance of formulation as expressing a version of events as recounted by another person and concurrently changing it (Heritage and Watson 1979, in Antaki 2008). It may be seen as politeness strategy, which explains why professionals sometimes seem to operate inefficiently and irrationally in interactions with clients (see Brown and Levinson 1978). Formulations may be indirect and insubstantial in order to prevent loss of face. Such formulations may be a good starting point for analysing social work interactions. We will enumerate the most relevant strategies:

- Mitigating the seriousness of the issue by using diminutives, for example a child welfare worker saying that things in the family might go *a little* different (van Nijnatten *et al.* 2001), by vagueness or by softening words (Linell and Bredmar 1996; Suoninen 1999).
- Placing critical comments in a positive context, for example giving optimistic news after bad tidings (Leydon 2008).
- Delay of introducing delicate issues or delicate terms (Weijts *et al.* 1993; Suoninen 1999).
- Expressing commonality between professional and client and down-playing possible conflicts (van Nijnatten 2007a).
- Indirectness and distancing by avoiding personal pronouns or names (depersonalisation, Weijts *et al.* 1993) or by using an institutional 'we' (Heritage and Maynard 2006), meta-language (van Nijnatten 2005) or humour (Norrick and Spitz 2008).
- Laughter (Haakana 2001) and smiling (Haakana 2010) as affiliative responses to prior remarks that were constructed as sensitive issues. Laughing may indicate that the one who is telling about a difficult issue is troubles-resistive, whereas the recipient shows troubles-receptiveness by not joining in this laughing (Jefferson 1984).
- Hedging by making disclaimers and pointing at future institutional decisions (Hutchby and Wooffitt 1998).
- The use of hypothetical questions may prepare the client for difficult issues that may have to be discussed in the future (Peräkylä 2005; Speer and Parsons 2006; Noordegraaf *et al.* 2008).

- Referring to the client as an experienced expert as a way to change the kind of relationship that clients and professionals have to the descriptions they report (indicated as 'footing' by Goffman (1981)).

Most of these interactional strategies are sequential and local, which is to say they are limited to special kinds of formulations that are used when potentially delicate issues are to be discussed, or specific sequences in the interaction.

Sequentiality

Sequentiality is an interactional strategy to deal with delicate issues in social work conversations. In the former paragraph, we have already discussed examples in which sequence plays a relevant role. Making disclaimers by referring to future decisions or expressing commonality before going into delicate topics are local strategies to manage conversations in which sensitive issues come up for discussion.

Next to these local strategies, sequentiality plays a crucial role in dealing with sensitivity over a longer stretch of talk, at the level of the whole session or a series of sessions (see Chapter 2). This strategy extends the direct dialogue and is based on the structure of the conversation in successive phases. This may include repeating a conversational strategy in successive phases. A pattern that is established while discussing non-sensitive issues may be used in sensitive parts of the conversation.

In all strategies of doing delicacy, it is relevant how professional and client respond to each other's expressions about the topics under discussion. These reactions may be estimated as a signal that the formulation is accepted (i.e. topic uptake) or rejected. Rejection itself can be understood as a delicate issue that necessitates delicacy marking. However, marking something as delicate can mean different things. It may refer to someone's personal style: some people speak less hesitantly than others. It would then be necessary to compare the differences in departures in a person's talk rather than the styles of separate persons. An additional difficulty is that not all perturbations arise from perceived delicacy, but may also be caused by someone searching through his/her memory or taking notes. In the end, what is essential in the construction of interaction is not what the speaker meant with the changes in the tone or style s/he used, but how the conversational partner interpreted those changes.

Doing delicacy in social work interaction: data examples and analyses

Two cases are presented to illustrate the use in practice of the methodological tools discussed above. Both cases are examples of institutional communication between a representative of a professional agency and a client. Both illustrate a special form of social work intervention because of the relation to the court. In both cases, the social worker has to prepare an enquiry for the court. It is relevant whether the client tells the truth about what happened and gives a complete image of his/her social and personal circumstances. We shall see in both cases that it is crucial that the social workers act with caution when issues in this sensitive context are (to be) discussed.

The way of analysing in the two cases is different. The first case aims at illustrating how much delicacy may be identified even in a very short piece of data. The second case extends this micro-analysis to longer interaction processes in which the organisational task is carried out.

Sensitivity of telling the truth

The first example is an episode of a conversation between a social worker (SW) of a Finnish probation agency and an 18-year-old client (C). The aim of this particular professional encounter is to obtain information about the client that is needed in order to write an assessment about the client's suitability to carry out his sentence, a short prison term, in *community service*. The assessment is important since it is one of the crucial documents on which the court will base its verdict. Because of the nature of the assessment it is essential that the social worker finds her client trustworthy.

The following data extract (a more detailed analysis is in Suoninen 1999) serves to illustrate the idea of identifying delicacy markers, because it includes many kinds of departures from everyday talk. The social worker seems to hint something very important without pronouncing it clearly. In order to make reading of the fragment easier the potentially delicate 'hot topic' is written with italic font.

Extract 1

1	SW:	In the assessment one does not n- does not need to
2		worry about crimes or anythi[ng
3	C:	[Yea
4	SW:	Whereas in the background information, on the other
5		hand, (.) it is permitted to (2) like for
6		example like if you look at this (.) summary then
7		there, (.) [it,
8	C:	[Yea
9	SW:	You <u>we</u>re judged guilty there in any case. (1)
10		Afterwards *I was wondering whether you were*
11		*fooling us* here or ( ) was the last heh an attempt
12		like to avoid (already) this matter ((after 'fooling
13		us' there is laughter up until now)) since it after all

14		stood in such a contradiction [to the record where
15	C:	[my-hy
16	SW:	You had confessed.hh but _that_ is an old story it
17		does not matter anymore.

What is marked as a delicate (or vexed or 'hot') issue is 'fooling us' in line 11. It is noteworthy how many features can be identified that may be understood as delicacy-marking devices. These include indirect word choices, perturbations, humour and explanations.

Soft word choices include many partly related aspects. First, the social worker chooses the softer term 'fooling us' rather than 'lying'. Second, instead of giving a proposition, advice or order (e.g. 'You lied to me' or 'Don't lie to me'), the social worker uses a question form. And, finally, instead of a simple question ('Did you lie to me?'), she uses a less certain clause ('I was wondering whether you were fooling us').

By this softened utterance the social worker avoids attributing a stigmatising identity category of unreliable person and thus saves the client's face.

Perturbations, which also make the 'fooling us' delicate, are situated before the mentioning of this hot topic. They consist of repetition ('does not n- does not', line 1), extra pauses, the use of 'like' twice and 'in any case' once in lines 5, 6 and 9, and a complicated search for the main point in lines 6, 7 and 9.

Humour and extra explanations occur after the potentially delicate hot topic. Speaking with laughter in one's voice is situated in lines 10–11. Humorous style may here serve two different functions. On the one hand, it may soften the critique by the social worker that the client was not honest. On the other hand, it may serve to save the face of the social worker herself because accusing someone else may also be understood as a delicate issue. As mentioned earlier, laughing may indicate that the one who is telling about difficulties is troubles-resistive (Jefferson 1984).

Extra explanations consist of the humorously uttered account and another one occurs after the potentially delicate hot topic. The first, an alternative humorous attempt at an account for 'fooling us', is situated just after this potentially delicate topic ('or was the last heh attempt like to avoid . . . this matter'. . ., lines 11–12), and the second in the last two lines ('But that is an old story it does not matter any more'). The last account that ends discussion of the topic serves to place critical comment in a positive context (Leydon 2008).

When looking at the responses of the client, it seems that, in spite of the potentially delicate issue that threatens the client's face, the interaction is jointly constructed. We can recognise this in his cooperative response ('mh-hy' in line 15) after the social worker's description. However, this response was not given immediately after the hot topic (lines 10–11) but only after the social worker's humorous talk, softening explanation and neutral description of facts.

From this short extract it is also possible to interpret the cues about categories that may be heard to be present in the social worker's speech. Although the hot topic is uttered in a soft way ('I was wondering whether you were fooling us'), it is possible to hear this expression as a category-bound activity hinting that the client belongs to the category of a 'liar' or 'untrustworthy person'. In spite of this category a very different one is hinted at just after this association, by saying with a laughing voice: 'or ( ) was the last heh an attempt like to avoid (already) this matter' (lines 11–12). Although difficult to hear as positive, this hints at a more understandable category of a rational if forgetful person, even if the social worker would not accept this kind of rationality in the future.

Doing delicacy in probation office work as illustrated above may serve many important functions as part of social work. When an issue is marked as delicate, it (here 'telling the truth') becomes distinctive from less important 'routine matters'. Doing delicacy also prevents 'turn-off' reactions in issues that may be felt to be hostile and thus maintains continuity and smoothness in conversation. It also creates a positive atmosphere for giving personal advice and hints.

Cautious building of an incest case

The second example shows the interaction between a social worker of the Dutch Child Protection Council (SW) and a stepfather (SF). The task of the Council is to assess family situations and report to the court if there are serious reasons to limit or remove parental authority. Prior to the conversation with SF, SW interviewed the mother of this family and one of her sons, Robin (see van Nijnatten 2013). The immediate cause for the Council's interference is a report from Robin's school in which serious problems are raised. SF and the mother are separated but the former frequently visits the family. The mother accuses SF of sexually abusing some of her children. The mother told SW that she is being treated for cancer and metastasis has been found, but SF doubts the seriousness of her condition. These extracts are about the interaction between SW and SF. In a previous interview, SW said that she was aware of both the seriousness of Robin's behaviour and the mother's accusations, which both pointed at the possibility of sexual abuse by SF. Yet she indicated that she was planning to start the conversation with SF with an open mind. She hoped to enable him to tell his story and so get more information about what was going on in the family.

In the beginning of the encounter, SW introduces Robin's toilet problems. SF takes the opportunity to show his caring responsibility for his stepson and the mother's lack of cooperation. Frequently he demonstrates his parental attentiveness and responsibilities, both as it is and in comparison with the mother. He stresses the mother's unwillingness to cooperate and

finally sighs that, in fact, he does not want to talk about her at all. The
fragment begins about ten minutes after the start of the interview (208).

Extract 2

215	SW:	Do you talk this ((mother's medical condition)) over with
216		the children?
217	SF:	Yes (.) when the children have a problem with that. For
218		example, when she goes completely out of her mind
219		again. Then I talk this over with the children and I
220		comforted them a little like: 'little man er your mother
221		might have cancer but in fact, at this point, I am sure
222		that she does not have it, because I spoke to the family
223		doctor (.) he didn't say much, I am not allowed to tell
224		the only thing he told me'. I wonder why she is in that
225		scooter. 'And secondly, when she had had cancer I
226		would have known'. That is clear for me. For me a clear
227		answer.
228	SW:	Yes in any case that is an answer
229	SF:	That is what I mean. He is not allowed to say anything
230		but for me that was quite a clear answer
231	SW:	Of course it is not unimportant to know
232	SF:	[and I am _very_ worried about that]
233	SW:	[for of it _is_ the case and and she//certainly when it is
234		so serious that she will die, then of course it is
235		important to discuss with each other where to go from
236		there]
237	SF:	Yes on the one side she says
238	SW:	You just said already in a firm tone 'then they come
239		with me'
240	SF:	Yes sure those two live already with me officially so I
241		get those with me at once
242	SW:	Yes

SW's reaction to SF's demonstration of his parental capabilities and his
imputation of the mother show that she does not agree but her formulation
is indirect with a double negation in turn 231. Although the social worker
does not fully agree, she starts her reaction in turn 217 with an affirmation.
This comforting strategy reinforces SF's conversational position. In turn 233,
SW again starts her turn with an affirmative word. She emphasises the
common ('each other') interest of SF and SW to discuss the children's future
situation. She avoids a confrontation about the mother's integrity, but
rather formulates it as relevant information for SF to have. This reading is

affirmed by SF at once (217), stressing his concern about the children. In the rest of the fragment, the interlocutors continue their positive and cooperative conversational style by starting their turn with 'Yes'. Although there might be opportunities for open conflict about this issue, both interlocutors succeed in constructing a positive interaction. While SF and SW talk at cross-purposes, SF describing his reactions to the mother's poor parenting and SW discussing the impact of the mother's illness on the children's future, their interaction bears the semblance of a cooperative conversation (van Nijnatten 2013).

In the next few minutes (fragment not shown), SF elaborates on his conversations with child welfare agencies and the family court. SW shows an attentive approach by commenting positively on SF's elaborations, by encouraging him to extend his narrative about his past experiences with child welfare and by putting his negative comments in perspective. In a smooth and natural-looking process (without special topic orientation markers, Fraser 2009), the topic of the conversation now has shifted to the children's condition. SW's style remains unchanged, asking about professional assessments, avoiding any discussion about the content of these, and reinforcing SF's elaborations. She uses connecting adverbs (for, and, because) rather than distancing adverbs (but, on the contrary, oh?). While continuing his narrative, SF follows a chronological and procedural order, at the same time revealing many details about the children's actual condition (see Chapter 6 on narrative).

SW introduces Robin's school report, starting with the report's positive feedback on the boy's performances, followed by an open question for SF's ideas about Robin's problems (opening a perspective-display series). SF thinks Robin's main problem is that he is soiling his pants. Although SW already knows about this, she lets SF give his version. In an unchanged style, SW asks neutral formulated questions, now focused on the children, followed by asking SF's opinion about this, emphasising that she is asking for his ideas rather than a report of the course of events. SW remains in her enquiry role and asks how SF is dealing now with the children's toilet problems.

Extract 3

894	SW:	Yes well regarding this soiling his pants, fairly often this
895		is connected with sexual abuse
896	SF:	Right
897	SW:	(.) Was this a point of discussion before or any cause
898	SF:	[Yes it was]
899	SW:	[to think this over?]
900	SF:	[for then there was this story that I would have sexually
901		abused him er Robin]
902	SW:	You would who??

```
903  SF:    So that I abused the children
904  SW:    All er Richard all so everybody?
905  SF:    Well yes euh, here in the walkway she was yelling and
906         you abused all my children. Well I got my hands on her
907         and I almost chucked her over the balcony (.) she may
908         have told you herself?
909  SW:    May be she did but there are such long periods
910         between the encounters
```

Now, SW relates the boys' toilet problems to sexual abuse. Her presentation is passive (895), indirect (897) and formulated as expertise (894). Avoiding any reference to SF himself, SW, in a kind of procedural format, asks whether this was ever brought up for contemplation. It is noteworthy that SF himself tells that he is under suspicion (900–901). SF's self-correction at the end of this turn is remarkable, indicating that the accusation may be interpreted more broadly. The next question of SW shows that SF's remark is a turning point in the interaction, SW asking SF to say more about the accusation that he would have abused more of the children. After this, SW changes her interview style into an interrogation format. In the following, SW says that the key question is whether anything has happened. SF then tells about a consultation with the family doctor who advised him about checking his sons' sexual hygiene. In a soft voice, SW reacts that that does not cause encropesis, hinting at a different cause of Robin's problem. This is the first, indirect and soft-voiced, accusation of SF by SW.

Extract 4

```
1004  SW:    Are you familiar with let's say this kind of problems say
1005         or or or?
1006  SF:    What do you mean?
1007  SW:    Well anyhow concerning sexual abuse you are accused
1008         now but that it occurs in the family or that you yourself
1009         . . .?
1010  SF:    Well I er the point is that I was abused from when I was
1011         fourteen
1012  SW:    Yourself?
1013  SF:    Yes my father was a war crimi/er victim of war
1014  SW:    [Yes]
1015  SF:    [who abused me.] And I was abused by a teacher from
1016         the Sunday school, at school I once was abused I went
1017         to [name place] by bike and I asked someone the road
1018         and er it went like: 'what would you like to drink', 'yes
1019         I'd like something to drink' and I ended up at the man's
1020         house
```

Now SW no longer avoids personal pronouns but uses 'problem' as a general category, which enables her to avoid a more specific and confronting term. By adding 'let's say' (line 1004) she informs SF that they (' let *us* say') will deliberately use mitigating terms. This is a special kind of delicacy marker, because it not only contains a softening metaphor but rather is a meta-remark revealing that softening metaphors are used in the conversation. The first lines of this fragment contain various delicacy markers, that is, the use of soft words ('problems', 'this kind of problems') followed by a demonstration of hesitation by 'or or or'. SF's reaction (1006) shows he is on his guard, demonstrating his awareness about the delicacy of the issue. In the next turn, SW takes up the accusation of abuse, but her approach remains cautious, using the passive voice ('are accused'), adding 'but' and offering two options for further discussions. Yet offering these options is also a subtle topic change, not challenging SF to react on the issue of the accusation. Indeed, SF takes the opportunity to describe his history of being abused as a child. After this extract, SW helps SF by putting the reported events in the perspective of a long past history. SW responds positively to SF's openness. Both conversation partners remain in an upward spiral of giving compliments and reinforcing each other's communicative intentions. This supports further the disclosure of SF.

Extract 5

1066	SW:	For in your idea there is a clear relation with the abuse
1067		the abuse you yourself experienced
1068	SF:	[Yes]
1069	SW:	[and by that in relationships with adults and children
1070		you yourself (?)?]
1071	SF:	I can talk about it more easily I learn that easily
1072	SW:	Yes you do talk (.) I mean quiet (.) calmly, I suppose
1073	SF:	Yes because I er yes just as I said the eldest child will
1074		have suffered most then (.) and probably he still suffers
1075		from it
1076	SW:	Her oldest child?
1077	SF:	Her her
1078	SW:	Her?
1079	SF:	Yes
1080	SW:	Those boys?
1081	SF:	Yes
1082	SW:	Yes
1083	SF:	[And then yes (. . . ? . . .)]
1084	SW:	[You said feeling up, you felt them up or did they (.)
1085		you? You asked if they (.)]
1086	SF:	No the children just slept with me and and and but the

```
1087            child touched me also and without force and once (.)
1088            again they were for me just two little human beings who
1089            were equal to me (.) and not so much the one
1090            dominating the other or whatever.
```

SW's open interview attitude incites SF to disclose, now giving crucial information about the actual sexual abuse of his stepchildren in guarded terms (lines 1086–1090). By using 'for in your idea' (1066), SW again uses a perspective-display series (Maynard 1991), describing the relation between SF's experiences as victim and perpetrator, as SF's construction. After a meta-exchange about SF's open approach and without any direct leading questions, SF's disclosure proceeds. It is telling that SF feels confident enough to return himself to this issue. This may also be the result of SW's praising remarks about SF's communicative performance. Like saying 'I mean' and 'I suppose', this is another marker of the delicacy of the issue under discussion.

After this extract, SF admits his attraction to his stepsons by telling that he is avoiding tempting situations. SW twice asks for confirmation of SF's disclosures and continues the enquiry mode by a new question. SF confirms that the problems decrease when the children become adolescents. Following this, SW makes a crucial step by touching the issue of incest. But again, she does so in an indirect way, by quoting SF's previous remark that he did not abuse the children ('And you say that nothing happened (.) between you and your children?'). This is followed by a hypothetical question ('If it was true (.) would you report?'), trying to get information about SF's approach while avoiding directly asking if SF *has* something to report. This type of question urges the other to answer the question (Noordegraaf *et al.* 2009).

Extract 6

```
1254  SW:    When you look at your children, would would you
1255         think that your children may have sexually abused
1256         probably? (.) You yourself has the experience
1257  SF:    Indeed I have
1258  SW:    [on both sides both as victim and as perpetrator]
1259  SF:    [Indeed I once wondered]
1260  SW:    You thought so, didn't you?
1261  SF:    Yes (.) after this soiling his pants
1262  SW:    Mm
1263  SF:    I do think that
1264  SW:    That is something we all think about don't we?
1265  SF:    Exactly that is what I thought myself
```

It is no surprise that the first direct dealing with the abuse did not lead to a confession. In order to establish that the children indeed were the victim of sexual abuse, SW addresses SF as an 'experience expert', who on the basis of his personal experiences may better know how to detect this in children's behavior (van Nijnatten 2007b).

She addresses him as both victim and offender. By formulating these two qualifications in one and the same breath it is less obvious that she is prompting a confession. It is relevant that SF does not use his turn to deny this qualification (1259). The social worker directly confirms SF's mental process, showing empathy, and reconstructs this semi-confession into an institutional conclusion by saying that it is something that 'we all' think about.

SW uses several conversational strategies to construct SF's confession of incest. As well as displaying caution in approaching the boy's toilet problems, SF's history of sexual abuse and his current involvement in Robin's life, she uses perspective-display series, asking SF's perspective, knowledge and views on the relevant issues (Maynard 1991). This is a step-by-step strategy to approach the issue of incest while taking SF's perspective into account. This of course may be considered a clever strategy to trap SF and to let him confess without openly asking him. Yet at the same time this may be seen as giving SF a chance to gradually come to the conclusion that he can no longer have uncontrolled parental authority over his stepchildren.

Implications for social work practice

In our illustrations it has been demonstrated that delicacy is the result of cautious lexical choice and interactional strategies. The strategies that were mentioned in the scientific literature in this field were found in the social work cases we presented. Social workers tried to avoid open conflicts with their clients by the use of cautious expressions, indirectness and avoidance. In other words, by their interactional performance, they prepared their clients to deal with sensitive issues. But this is only half of the story. Doing delicacy is not just the work of professionals in relation to their clients, it has an interactional result, clients and professionals cooperating to find a way to pass off the interaction smoothly. Moreover, people do not enter interactions with others unprepared. They have expectations about the other participants in the interactions and ideas about the setting of the communications. Tannen and Wallat (1987) use the concept of 'knowledge schema' for pre-situational expectations that, together with frames, are conditional for interactions. Yet how expectations work out in the communication between participants can only be analysed by looking at the actual conversation.

The court relatedness and the client's expertise with former service provision might be enough reason to freeze the conversations in the two cases. Yet such a prediction does not reckon with the dynamics of the interactions between social workers and clients. In both cases, the professional succeeded in preventing open conflict and in the second case this led to information that was crucial for the social worker's assessment. We have shown that, even if some issues are assessed beforehand as strongly sensitive, even taboo, social workers and their clients have many strategies at their disposal to construct them as normal enough to be discussed without too much morality. Doing delicacy in social work is securing an interactional space in order to enable progress with regard to the institutional goals 'behind' the conversation. By treating issues with respect for the client's sensitivities, professionals try to secure their cooperation and to increase client sincerity.

Moreover, this chapter shows that 'doing delicacy' is not limited to local sequences in the conversations but rather extends to the construction of an argumentation on the level of the whole encounter. In the second case, it is illustrated that the social worker brought about a crucial confession that is needed for an assessment, by constructing a case in separate and gradual steps. She did so by first paying attention to the mother's and SF's parenting tasks, establishing a relation between the boys' toilet problems and child abuse, and finally to SF's possible involvement in the abuse. It is remarkable that the social worker did little more than follow a procedure with a seemingly natural chronological order. But this procedure was accompanied by repeated positive remarks that made the client feel comfortable. This enabled the client to introduce crucial topics. By following this procedure, the social worker succeeded in going from daily parenting problems to the client's possible involvement in incest. The procedure is the combination of a strict neutral question format and a repeated positive reinforcement of the client's conversational contributions. The strategy resembles the therapeutic strategy of systematic desensitisation, introducing issues at a higher and higher level of stress, followed at each level by comforting the client. By acting this way, the social worker succeeded in getting closer and closer to the client's complete disclosure of a most delicate secret. This procedure may be seen as an effective strategy to secure confessions in complex and sensitive cases, but at the same time this process of gradualness may be seen as a prudent professional strategy in which clients, in spite of their irresponsible behaviour, are approached with respect. The analysis of the transcript of a whole session allowed us to show how the management of delicacy is spread out over the whole interaction and consists of successive steps in which a case is built (compare Komter 2003).

Social work is directed at daily social problems of citizens and is located in the semipublic sector of society. It is involved in the new relationship between public and private that, at the end of the nineteenth century, emerged in most western societies. Social work belongs to the midfield of society that is involved with problems of poverty, hygiene, education and sexuality. Social work is engaged in the private life of families and individuals. In their daily work, social workers are confronted with dilemmas between autonomy and control, responsiveness and standardisation, and demand and supply. They may assess if elderly people can maintain their independent way of life or rather have to be taken into elderly care, they may meet unemployed people who are required to do more job interviews on penalty of a reduction in benefit, or they may talk to parents of families at risk who have to raise their children differently on pain of losing their parental authority. They may also work with delinquents looking for rehabilitation, or individuals at risk who want to regain their authority to act. Social workers communicate with people in danger and/or dangerous people (Donzelot 1979). This type of institutional communication is often seen as especially difficult, because the social worker has to provide the client with sad, negative or otherwise confronting information, or because it is the professional's task to obtain delicate information from the client.

Hence, 'doing delicacy' seems an everyday occurrence in social work. When an issue is marked as delicate, it becomes important because of its distinction from unproblematic matters. In addition, doing delicacy prevents the silencing of discussion in issues that may be felt to be threatening (psychological level) and thus maintains continuity and smoothness in conversation (interactional level). It creates a positive atmosphere, on the one hand, for giving personal advice and hints and, on the other hand, for making disclosures. In addition it contributes in turning important practices into a self-evident local culture, and thus building a long-term professional–client relation.

Social work is brought into action when individuals or groups are at odds with societal norms. Its strategies are often sophisticated ways of changing clients' behaviour in an effort to align clients' conduct and social standards. Dealing with sensitive issues is a crucial element in these strategies as it is focused on sensitive issues, which accompany the problems at stake. In this perspective, features of speech that are discussed above are often relevant actions to achieve the social work goal. They constitute an essential part of professional skill rather than a 'disturbance' that may be an indication of lack of professional routine.

10

REPORTED SPEECH

Kirsi Juhila, Arja Jokinen and Sirpa Saario

Social work conversations are usually rich with talk about past events and encounters. In professional–client discussions clients might describe incidents with their family members or visits to a health care centre. Additionally, in meetings among professionals, participants can inform each other about situations or the behaviour of clients that they have recently met. This kind of talk about the past is commonly done by reporting what other people or the narrator said in a described situation. In other words, past voices are brought into conversations. This can be seen in professional–client conversations: 'My husband said to me that I have looked very tired over the last few weeks', 'The doctor assumed that I might suffer from depression.' It can also be seen in meetings among professionals: 'Maria (the client) said she cannot afford to pay her rent', 'Erik (the client) was very angry yesterday and swore at me, saying you are a bloody idiot.' These kinds of past voices used in conversations are called *reported speech* and in this chapter we shall look at its use in social work interaction.

As the previous brief examples demonstrate, reported speech is an integral element of social work talk. It is naturally not only typical of social work but is common in all kinds of talk where people meet each other and talk about their or other people's news or experiences, or about events and incidents they have been involved in. As Bakhtin (1981: 337) states: 'The transmission and assessment of the speech of others, the discourse of another, is one of the most widespread and fundamental topics of human speech.' In spite of this commonality, we seldom pay special attention to this feature of talk or call it reported speech.

Since social work conversations are professional, institutional forms of talk with certain tasks and purposes, and because social work so often focuses on people's problems and situations that have 'a past history', prior talk by different stakeholders is often brought into conversations. To return to our examples above, past voices can, for instance, have a significant part to play when deciding whether problems exist, how serious they are and what kinds of treatment and interventions are needed: whether the tiredness of the mother is regarded as a real mental health problem to be taken into account when planning child protection plans, whether clients are assessed as needing financial help, or whether clients are defined as 'badly behaving problem cases' that deserve certain disciplinary consequences. This chapter examines the richness and consequential nature of reported speech in social work interaction and provides tools to analyse it.

The functions of reported speech in social work interaction

In what follows, we first deepen the definition of reported speech and its origin in research. Then we deal with four relevant functions of reported speech in social work interaction and the ways to analyse them: producing evidence, constructing categorisations, assessing and accounting, and making narratives. The functions are often interwoven in interaction. The grouping of four functions is based on the review of such previous reported speech studies that have concentrated on analysing reported speech embedded in conversations. Although there is not much literature focusing especially on reported speech in social work interaction, we draw upon such writings that are relevant from the point of view of social work. After presenting the functions of reported speech, we proceed to analyse data examples from Finnish mental health and family violence work to illustrate the functions.

Reported speech and context

Studies focusing on reported speech in conversations often trace back the concept of reported speech to Bakhtin's (1981), Volosinov's (1971) and also to Goffman's (1981) work. The uses and functions of it have been studied across several disciplines, including linguistics, narrative and literary theory, sociology and philosophy (Holt 1996: 221; Stokoe and Edwards 2007: 335). Reported speech as an interactional accomplishment has been examined in ethnomethodology, conversation analysis, narrative approaches and discursive psychology. In this chapter we primarily make use of ethnomethodologically oriented studies on reported speech in face-to-face interaction, especially in institutional interaction (e.g. Baynham and Slembrouck 1999; Buttny 2004; Holt and Clift 2007; Tannen 2007).

Above we wrote that reported speech means past voices that are brought into conversations. To put this preliminary description more precisely, and following Buttny's (1998: 48) work, we define reported speech as *prior talk that is 'used and put into context in a present conversation'*. Reported speech can be *direct* or *indirect*, although these are often difficult to differentiate (Coulmas 1986; Holt 2000: 427–432). Direct reported speech means talk where the speaker seems to reproduce the actual/real words of the original speaker (e.g. 'Erik was very angry yesterday and swore at me, saying you are a bloody idiot'). Indirect reported speech takes the form of a summary of former utterances and sometimes also of ideas and thoughts composed by the teller without repeating the actual words (e.g. 'the doctor assumed that I might suffer from depression') (Coulmas 1986: 2–3; Holt 1996: 220–221; Buttny 1998: 48; Buttny 2004: 97).

In Buttny's definition of reported speech the concept of context is essential. Since reported speech is used in present talk, *the reporting context* is a crucial element in analysing the meanings and functions of it. It is not possible to divorce the context of reported speech and reporting from one another (Volosinov 1971: 153; Holt 1996: 222). Reported speech is always recontextualised: past voices are altered when reporting speakers use them for the purposes of the present context (Buttny 1998: 48–49). Volosinov (1971: 151) writes: 'There are, of course, essential differences between an active reception of another's speech and its transmission in a bound context.' So, although quoting original speakers creates the impression of authenticity, reported speech is not a disinterested report of events but is used to fulfil some tasks in the current interaction (Holt 1996: 221). This is important to recognise when studying reported speech in different social work contexts with various institutional agendas. For instance, the purposes of using clients' prior talk can be very different in a child abuse enquiry than in therapeutically oriented alcohol treatment. In the first case it can be used as a proof of abusive behaviour ('the father said to me that pulling children's hair is not violence but that it is sometimes a necessary part of responsible parenthood'). In the second case it might be in the service of a healing process ('do you remember the phase when you constantly told me that you didn't have problems with alcohol?').

Producing evidence

Much research has characterised reported speech as an economical and effective way of producing evidence (Wooffitt 1992; Holt 1996: 225–226; Stokoe and Edwards 2007: 335). Evidence production can be said to be the core interactional task of using reported speech, since almost all reported speech has this function (Myers 1999: 386). Using prior voices of others or oneself serves the task of presenting the described issues, state of affairs or events as accurate and factual.

The use of reported speech makes the reporting speaker's talk sound accurate and reliable because it distances the speaker from the message. By reporting the words and sentences that other people have said, speakers are able to describe how certain occasions have unfolded or what some states of affairs are like without making any interpretations of their own or regardless of their own points of view. For instance, Wooffitt (1992: 161–164) has analysed how speakers produce evidence of the objectivity of unexpected paranormal phenomena they have experienced not just by describing the prior phenomenon in the case, but also by reporting the words of others who witnessed the same phenomenon (e.g. 'my husband said my God what is it?'). This way of factual accounting or reporting is common in many social work interactions. When describing encounters with clients in their case notes, social workers can report direct or indirect quotations of clients or themselves and simultaneously produce evidence, for instance about cooperative or uncooperative clients, without explicitly using these evaluative categorisations. Clients can describe their previous behaviour, possibly assessed as non-desirable, to social workers by reporting the words of others: 'The passer-by said that he saw the other guy, not me, starting the fight.' In this last example a speaker presents a quotation to provide evidence for a potentially controversial issue; reported speech argues against the anticipated interpretation that the client might have been the originator of the fight. Likewise, social workers might use reported speech to convey the factuality of some state of affairs concerning clients with whom they themselves have been involved: in a meeting with colleagues a social worker might say that 'the doctor mentioned that he has also recognised how tired the mother was' when discussing the situation of a child welfare client and her need for supportive measures.

Reporting the words of an authority is often regarded as a very effective way to provide evidence and construct facts (Potter 1996: 114). For instance, in the previous example the social worker quotes the doctor, who is an expert in diagnosing people's physical well-being, and thus his/her direct words construct the mother's tiredness as a fact. The prior talk of those who have personal experiences related to the discussed issues or events can also be considered words of authority: 'The nurse who had met the client at several home visits said that his drinking problem has become worse', 'The woman living in the old people's home called and reported that the shortage of nursing staff has reduced the quality of the services there.'

As we mentioned at the beginning of this section, reported speech and evidence production are almost always connected to each other. When and how reported speech provides evidence is to be read only from the interactional dynamics of reporting contexts, where prior talk is always recontextualised. For instance, whose words are taken as the words of authority depends on the reporting context; sometimes reporting the woman's call from the old people's home can serve as evidence of clients complaining 'without proper reasons' rather than as evidence of bad service practices. So, in reporting contexts, the task of producing evidence is often linked to other functions of reported speech, such as categorisation and assessment. We now turn to discuss these functions.

Constructing categorisations

Previous research has shown that one function of reported speech is to create portraits or produce the characters of others (Hall *et al.* 1999; Buttny 2004). Using the words of others can thus be said to construct identity categorisations (see Chapter 3) by characterising the quoted persons in a certain light based on their prior talk. In the following extract a mother (M) answers a social worker's (SW) question about how she and her son are feeling at the moment at the beginning of a home visit (the example is from Hall *et al.* 2006: 77–79):

```
1    M:    Nathan was a bit upset when he came back the other day erm
2    SW:   from contact (.) is that with (father)
3    M:    erm yeah he said erm that he was upset because his dad
4          wouldn't listen to him (.) he's told him that he'd buy him
5          complete school uniform
6    SW:   hmm
7    M:    and he got upset because he insisted on buying him a (laugh)
8          pair of school trousers
9    SW:   hmm
10   M:    and he must've carried on saying that he didn't want it and he
11         got upset because his dad wouldn't listen to him and he said
12         you've got to have proper school trousers erm (.) and the
13         other
14   SW:   was that on Saturday Danielle
15   M:    yeah that was on Saturday
16   SW:   right
17   M:    and the other little thing was when he cooked him a dinner he
18         said that he wanted (laugh) mushrooms and his dad said you
19         don't like mushrooms and Nathan said yes I do but apart
20         from that it was ok
```

There is a lot of interactional business going on in this talk that we comment on later in this chapter. But looking at the portraits that the mother produces in collaboration with the social worker of two absent people – the son, Nathan, and his father – it is noticeable how their prior speech plays a significant role in this production. Hall *et al.* (2006: 78–79) write: 'we see a differentiation between the children and the father as elements of the family, the first sensitive and dependent and the second insensitive and excluded'. The father is constructed as a 'not listening' and deficient parent, while the mother presents herself as a sensitive and competent parent. The mother makes these categorisations 'true' (cf. produces evidence with reported speech) by reporting the tense, and thus concerning, conversation between the son and the father as it was told to her by Nathan. Noteworthy in this example is that creating portraits of others using reported speech is often simultaneously in the service of creating a person's self-categorisation. Commenting on others' prior speech displays discursive positioning of both others and oneself (Davies and Harré 1990; Buttny 2004: 98). Alternatively, as Holt (2000: 438) puts it: 'speech can convey both the attitude of the reported speaker and, more implicitly, the attitude of the current speaker'.

Portraits of others created by using reported speech can be employed to produce stereotyping categorisations. Buttny (1997, 2004; Buttny and Williams 2000) has examined in a series of studies how (prejudicial) race categorisation is done with reported speech among American students in informal campus talk. In one of Buttny's extracts (2004: 118) a White male says:

> a Black girl said to me last year that uhm she hangs out only with Black people because she chooses to she gets along with Black people better than White people and in general she doesn't like White people and I've heard a lot of White people say the same thing about Black people.

Buttny (2004: 118) states that when the reporting speaker quotes here what 'a Black girl said', he uses and treats it as evidence of the intergroup differences between Black and White people, an interpretation that he confirms with a summarising quote of a White person's prior talk. This kind of stereotyping – using culturally easily recognised categorisations – is familiar in many social work contexts and it is thus worth paying attention to how they might be reproduced by employing reported speech.

Using the words of others can create negative portraits of the quoted persons and possibly also of the category group they are associated with (negative stereotypes). Reported speech can make quoted persons sound stupid, ridiculous, unmoral, unreliable, incapable and so on (Buttny 2004: 105–106; Stokoe and Edwards 2007). Accordingly, as an action reported speech can be mocking, insulting, judging or discrediting, for example. Alternatively, creating positive categorisations of others by using reported speech is equally possible. Both kinds of categorisations are highly relevant when studying social work interaction (Hall *et al.* 1999) and, as Buttny (2004: 114) remarks, reported speech can also be a resource allowing the reporting speaker to resist, criticise and challenge negative portraits and stereotypes (see Chapter 8).

Creating negative and positive portraits, as well as resistance towards certain categorisations through quoting prior talk, links closely to the third function of reported speech, namely assessing and accounting.

Assessing and accounting

Reported speech has been shown to be connected to assessment in many ways (Holt 2000; Buttny 2004: 96; Couper-Kuhlen 2007). Furthermore, in instances where reporting speakers 'just' seem to repeat accurately what other speakers or they themselves have said on the described occasion, they can implicitly comment on reported utterances and thus simultaneously convey their assessment of reported talk (Holt 2000). As Buttny (2004: 146) writes, the studies have demonstrated how reporting speakers can frame the prior talk through negative or positive evaluation, presenting it in unfavourable or favourable light. Producing negative and positive assessments is usually linked to the creation of negative and positive portraits (categorisations) of reported people. It also associates closely with the production of factual evidence, since reported speech serves as evidence to support the assessment.

To return to the extract of the mother–social worker conversation, we can identify a strong sense of assessment in it. With the support of the social worker, the mother presents the father's behaviour as unfavourable by quoting his son's prior talk and the son's quotes of the father's prior talk in a certain negative framework. The reported speech can be said to do the complaining in the extract. Using reported speech in this way is widely recognised in previous studies (e.g. Günthner 1997; Drew 1998; Holt 2000; Haakana 2007; Stokoe and Edwards 2007). Haakana (2007: 154), who has studied reported thought in complaint stories, notes that complaints are typically about a quoted third party, who is not present in the reporting context. The talk of this absent party is then quoted to people who were not present in the original quoted situation. For instance, Stokoe and Edwards (2007) show how callers to UK neighbourhood mediation centres use reported speech, especially quoted racial insults, as one means of constructing complaints about their neighbours. So, in these calls the callers (or clients) quote absent neighbours' prior talk and present it to the mediators, who were not present in the reported situations. This kind of complaining talk about third parties is common in different social work settings. Both clients and social workers are continually quoting absent people in this kind of negative assessment framework.

Negative evaluation with the help of reported speech can also serve functions other than just complaining, for instance presenting the quoted persons and/or their behaviour as ridiculous and not to be taken seriously. When researching social work interaction the positive evaluations made with reported speech should not be forgotten either. As an example, social workers can discuss absent clients in a favourable light by using clients' prior talk as evidence of their positive assessments. Also clients can quote advice they received from social workers which respects and shows strong agreement with assessments' content. Another interesting aspect of reported speech related to assessment not to be overlooked is self-quoting and quoting the prior talk of people present in the reporting context. When encountering each other, clients and social workers easily report their former talk in the series of past encounters and make assessments, for instance of clients' progress or regression, through such speech.

When reported speech displays assessment it is often entangled with accounting, implicating discussions related to responsibilities, blame, excuses and justifications (Scott and Lyman 1968; see Chapter 4). Reported speech can be used as a means of producing, denying and accepting responsibility. Clients' calls to neighbourhood mediation centres, analysed by Stokoe and Edwards (2007), contain plenty of responsibility talk linked to reported talk. For instance, the neighbours' quoted racial insults are presented as one type of trouble with the neighbours, and simultaneously the neighbours are constructed as partly responsible for the disputes. The denial of the reporting speakers' own responsibility (and excusing or justifying one's own conduct in the reported context) by allocating blame to others might thus be one function of reported speech. However, the function can also be the opposite, for instance when clients quote their own prior talk in a negative light (self-blaming). When researching social work interaction attention should also be paid to how social workers use reported speech when accounting for their own or clients' former behaviour on various occasions.

As Holt (2000: 451) reminds us, assessments are done jointly in a reporting context:

> rather than making their assessment of the event explicit, reported speech (within a sequence containing implicit assessment) can be used to give the recipient the access to the utterance in question, thus allowing him or her to react to it and the teller to then collaborate in that reaction.

This is an important reminder when analysing social work interaction. Responses to quoted talk play an important part in assessment making. For instance, without the agreeing responses of the social worker in the extract presented earlier, the mother's complaining narrative based on the son's reported talk about the conduct of the father would not have been successful or become shared by the parties. As is the case in this example, assessing and accounting, as well as the evidence producing and categorisation related to them, are often presented in a narrative format. Making a narrative is the function of reported talk we look at more closely next.

Making narratives

Reported speech commonly occurs in a story form or embedded in narratives (Buttny 1998: 48–49), where events are narrated in chronological order and participants in these events are presented as story-world portraits (Couper-Kuhlen 2007: 81; see, in this book, Chapter 6). As Couper-Kuhlen (2007) notes, most previous research has concentrated on prior talk used in a story framework or in larger narrative contexts, although reported speech can also be produced in non-narrative frames. Reported speech is a resource people draw on in narratives, but simultaneously is also a means to make narratives. Buttny (1998: 49) states that reported speech often seems to capture the most crucial parts of a narrative.

Turning to the mother's description of her son Nathan's and his father's relationship, Hall *et al.* (2006: 78) demonstrate how the first part of it is presented in a storytelling framework:

> It is a complete story (Labov and Waletzky 1967) with an abstract (he was upset because his father wouldn't listen to him), orientation (dad promised a school uniform), complication (only bought him trousers and Nathan didn't want these trousers), resolution (father insisted on these trousers), and evaluation (father wouldn't listen to him).

This chronological story of how Nathan got upset draws heavily on the prior talk by the story figures (the father and Nathan), which forms the most crucial resource in narrative making. Quotes make the story vivid and convincing.

A common way to make narratives is to report the sequences of turns of the prior interaction (Holt 1996) or, in other words, to make narratives by constructing conversations between the characters in reported contexts (Tannen 2007). The mother's story described above is mainly based on the reported conversations between the father and Nathan. But it also includes another reported conversation, namely the one between the mother and Nathan: Nathan reported the conversations with his father to his mother, who now reports both of these conversations to the social worker. It is very usual that the reporting speakers describe their own prior conversations to third parties who were not present in the 'original' reported context. In our example the third party is the social worker in the context of an institutional home visit, to whom the mother describes the past conversations that occurred in non-institutional, family-life contexts. These kinds of reported conversations are typical in social worker–client interaction, but reported conversations are present in social work talk in many other ways as well, for instance when social workers report to each other their prior conversations with clients in a story form (Juhila *et al.* 2011).

Making narratives through reported speech in social work interaction is highly consequential. As with reported speech in general, it is used for providing evidence about past events, but more importantly it can be used as reporting the stances of the speakers as displayed in their talk (Holt 2000: 232). The presented stances give the grounds for making assessments of the speakers' attitudes, wrong-doings and right-doings in the reported context. Assessments and categorisations are often bound together, for example an uncaring father, an indifferent social worker or a motivated and well-progressed client. However, what should be remembered when analysing narratives containing reported talk and conversations is that the reporting context and its *in situ* conversation are always essential. Reporting speakers and the recipients of or listeners to reports create the story and produce its consequences in collaboration.

Reported speech in social work interaction: data examples and analyses

Next we will move on to analyse the accomplishment of four functions of reported speech in naturally occurring social work interaction. Our data are located in two different Finnish institutions and in two different conversational situations (reporting contexts). In the first example, two professionals discuss the situation and condition of the client. The client is not physically present in the interaction, but the professionals still use her voice a lot. This conversation between the professionals takes place in a mental health NGO (non-governmental organisation). In the second example, a professional and a client discuss the client's personal change process – her successful breakaway from a violent relationship. In this discussion, which takes place in a shelter targeted at people suffering from domestic violence, the client's own prior talk and the past conversations (reported conversations) between the professional and the client are used as resources in producing a progressive narrative.

Professional–professional conversation in a mental health NGO

Here, we consider the reported speech that takes place in the conversation between two professionals of a project established by a Finnish mental health NGO. The project carries out intensive rehabilitation courses for young people with severe mental health problems. The aim of the three-month courses is to intensify community-based rehabilitation by promoting clients' individual rehabilitation in various ways, for example by supporting and assessing their daily skills and their cognitive and social abilities. The conversation between the two professionals, presented in the following extract, takes place in a team meeting of the course's professionals. In these weekly meetings the professionals discuss the condition, behaviour and situation of the clients, and inform each other about the last week's events and incidents in the course.

The following conversation concerns a client called Julia. Previously, professionals have been talking about Julia's injured leg and how it might affect her participation in various rehabilitation activities. They now turn to discussion of Julia's mental health. P1, as Julia's keyworker, opens this topic (arrows in the extract indicate reported speech).

Extract 1

1		P1:	we have checked once a week how to follow her warning signs ((of
2			mental illness)) and [their seriousness
3		P2:	[yeah and something has emerged from it
4		P1:	yes and then I noticed she has not recorded at least in these ((follow-
5	→		up documents made by the client)) that when she once said in
6	→		her individual assessment conversation that she has every now and
7	→		then such feelings of anxiety that she feels [aggressive
8		P2:	[oh really
9	→	P1:	and something starts to irritate her so she gets such an aggressive
10	→		feeling [then that that
11		P2:	[erm
12	→	P1:	there are erm (.) voices [and and anxiety that might come
13		P2:	[erm
14		P1:	however she has not documented them in any way (.) here (.) but
15	→		I feel that it was also somehow such a delicate [topic for her that
16		P2:	[erm
17	→	P1:	even though she was able to say it [she didn't want to say anything
18		P2:	[yeah
19	→	P1:	after that [to process or discuss it any more
20		P2:	[yes yes yes yes but it is rather good that she has said it out
21			loud [that kind of thing
22		P1:	[yeah
23		P2:	anyway probably she doesn't open up so easily
24	→	P1:	and there was talk about whether she feels that they are those daily
25	→		[issues that do those voices appear daily and so on
26		P2:	[erm
27	→	P1:	[she replied that they don't appear daily
28		P2:	[erm
29	→	P1:	[but every now and then [now some weeks ago there had for
30		P2:	[erm [erm
31	→	P1:	instance been such a situation in a supermarket that she had act in
32	→		she suddenly got an unreal feeling and then she couldn't do the
33	→		shopping that she had planned beforehand [I said that how did you
34		P2:	[yeah yeah
35	→	P1:	that situation [that did you go away from the store [did you interrupt
36		P2:	[erm [mm
37	→	P1:	everything that you were doing so she said that she just thought
38	→		that she can make some purchases and then goes away but [then
39		P2:	[erm
40	→	P1:	she couldn't however do those things that she had thought about
41	→		beforehand [(1) but these things don't happen often she says but
42		P2:	[yeah yeah

43		P1:	she isn't like that at least now according to this monitoring [so
44		P2:	[yeah
45		P1:	so she hasn't withdrawn anything ((referring to withdrawing money
46			from an account))
47		P2:	yes yes (3)
48		P?:	°yeah° (2)
49		P1:	and she really doesn't have that many coping skills [that
50		P2:	[erm
51	→	P1:	she said that she is not able to in a way to calm down to read or
52	→		anything that then when [she gets in to that kind of state of anxiety
53		P2:	[yeah
54	→	P1:	she can't think of anything other than taking medicine then [(.)and
55		P2:	[yeah
56		P1:	she has also taken it here
57		P2:	yeah (2) erm (3)
58		P1:	but she is probably also such the type who doesn't talk so honestly [talk
59		P2:	[erm
60		P1:	about her own feelings looks good on the surface but then
61	→	P2:	yes you can somehow see it that when you look at her she said for instance
62	→		today at the morning meeting that she is ok but somehow
63		P1:	erm
64	→	P2:	and it is exactly same with Jake he also might say that he is doing
65	→		pretty ok
66		P1:	erm
67		P2:	but somehow you notice from their appearance or how they say it
68		P1:	yeah
69		P2:	so you notice that they are not ok but something (else)

The above dialogue is rich in reported speech. Both professionals (P1 and P2) act as reporting speakers. P1 is the main reporting speaker, whereas P2 only quotes the previous talk of the client at the end of the extract (lines 61–62). The quoted speakers are the client, Julia and P1, the professional who is also the main reporting speaker and who thus quotes herself. Also, in the last turn of P2, another client, Jake, is quoted. The example includes direct reported speech (e.g. lines 33–37), indirect reported speech including reported thought (e.g. lines 5–7, 15 and 17), and reported conversations (e.g. 24–41).

Reported speech is used strongly for producing evidence that the client is not in a very good state when it comes to her mental health. The factuality of this state of affairs is made above all by quoting the client herself (see Smith 1978). In the beginning, P1 reports the speech of the client by saying that, in their private conversations, Julia said that at times she suffers from states of anxiety, she feels aggressive and gets irritated, and that voices may emerge (lines 4–12). P1 confirms this further by describing a conversation in which she and Julia talked about how Julia failed to do everyday errands (to complete the shopping) due to 'unreal feeling' (lines 29–40). The client's prior words, reported internal experiences about her mental health, serve here as words of authority. Moreover, P1's own role in past conversations also presents words of authority. As the client's keyworker she has been close to her and thus owns reliable information about her condition: P1 reports the content of individual conversations between herself and the client and her own 'fact-seeking' questions posed for the client to answer (lines 5–12, 24–41).

By using reported speech the professionals create a certain portrait or an identity categorisation for an absent third party, Julia. As we already demonstrated above, she is portrayed as a client with some mental health problems (having feelings of anxiety, aggressiveness and irritation, and hearing voices), which is not a surprise when taking account of the reporting context. However, by quoting the client's past talk and thoughts P1 adds a further dimension to this categorisation (lines 14–19). Julia is the kind of person who does not open up easily about her mental state: 'she didn't want to say anything after that to process or discuss it any more' (lines 17 and 19). Later, P1 continues this 'not opening up easily' categorisation by identifying Julia as one of those types who 'doesn't talk so honestly' (line 58). P2 recognises this stereotype of clients immediately and confirms the idea that Julia belongs to this group of clients by reporting Julia's prior talk (she said that 'she is ok') and its discrepancy with her appearance (lines 60–62). She also provides further evidence that this type of client group really exists by quoting Jake and then commenting on a general level about the discrepancy between the 'ok talk' of these clients and their appearances (lines 64–69). It is noteworthy that not only the clients but also the professionals themselves are categorised through reported speech in the example. When quoting their own prior talk from conversations with the clients, P1 and P2 portray themselves as mental health professionals, who have discussions with the clients and who observe and assess them in various settings.

Assessment and reported speech are firmly connected to each other in this conversation between two professionals. As we already pointed out, the client's prior talk is framed with a negative evaluation (with a 'complaining' tone) in the sense that she is categorised as a person who is not willing to talk further about her problems. However, P2 mitigates this categorisation when she comments on the reported conversation presented by P1: 'but it is rather good that she has said it out loud anyway probably she doesn't open up so easily' (lines 20–23). This positive evaluation based on the client's reported speech produces the prospect that Julia's recovery process is possibly off to a good start. Though really, at a good start only, there is still a lot to do. This kind of assessment is made evident, again with the help of the client's own previous talk: 'she said that she is not able to in a way to calm down to read or anything that then when she gets in to that kind of state of anxiety she can't think of anything other than taking medicine then' (lines 51–54). By reporting this speech, Julia is assessed as not fully coping with her illness since the only coping skill she has is to resort to medicine.

In spite of the assessment that Julia has not progressed very far in her recovery, the tone of the conversation is not a blaming one. Julia's voice is quoted in an understanding manner and treated partly as accounts excusing her behaviour. For instance, her story about the incident in the store includes an excuse: because of her 'unreal feeling' she was not able to finish her shopping as planned, but she did what she was able to in a difficult situation (lines 29–41). All in all, Julia's own prior talk is mainly presented as authoritative talk in itself, such as her 'diagnosis' of this store incident, of her feelings (lines 5–12), of her difficulties in processing her feelings further (lines 14–19) or of her limited coping skills (lines 51–54). However, there are also elements of anticipated blame and responsibility present in a sense that, in the next step of the recovery process, the client should be more active in disclosing honestly her inner feelings to the professionals (lines 58–60).

As is usual, reported speech occurs in this example in narratives. The example includes several short narratives that are in the service of producing evidence, categorisation and assessment. The short narratives in particular are made by reporting the sequences of turns of the prior interactions in which the professionals and the absent client had participated. These reported conversations include the individual assessment conversation (lines 5–19), the discussion relating to the store incident embedded in the assessment conversation (lines 24–41) and the very short encounter during the morning meeting (lines 61–65).

A social worker–client conversation in a shelter targeted at people suffering from domestic violence

The following conversation takes place at a Finnish shelter for individuals or families who have experienced or been threatened with domestic violence. The participants are a social worker and a young female client, Lisa, who has stayed at the shelter with her two small children for about a month. During her time there, she has come to the conclusion that she will not return to her husband and she is moving into a new home with her children the following day. The conversation thus deals with the ending of her clienthood.

Before the following data extract, the social worker and the client have reviewed the client's life, which had been full of violence, and talked about how her life has gradually taken a turn for the better during her stay at the shelter. Lisa has been very open about her feelings concerning the violent situations she has experienced, and she has said that she is looking forward to moving into a flat of her own. In the extract, the social worker makes an evaluative summary of the process the client has gone through, using Lisa's reported speech. Thus, the example describes the use of prior talk by a person who is present in a situation where the reporting speaker (the social worker, SW) and the reported speaker (the client, C) are engaged in a conversation (arrows in the extract indicate reported speech).

Extract 2

1	→	SW:	what I think is really imp<u>o</u>rtant to see is what you <u>said</u> just a moment
2	→		ago (.) oh better check if the tape's about to run out
3		C:	((laughter))
4	→	SW:	what you <u>said</u> just now I mean you said (3) ((sounds of dealing with tape
5			recorder))
6		C:	now it is r<u>un</u>[ning ok
7		SW:	[good ((sounds of dealing with tape recorder, laughter))
8			the <u>thing</u> you.hhhh (.) that <u>when</u> (.) when you were in ((mentions name
9			of home town)) (.) and you (.) saw him (.) <u>La</u>sse there (.) when you
10	→		turned to l<u>oo</u>k (.) and you thought I'm going to (.)
11		C:	ye[es (I'm)
12	→	SW:	[I'm <u>going</u> to die he[re
13		C:	[ye-[es
14	→	SW:	[like this is the last moment of my <u>life</u>.hhhhh
15			so that's where you <u>started</u> that was <u>sort</u> of the <u>worst</u> poi[nt
16		C:	[that was the
17			wor[st that was [maybe what it's (.) .h[hh
18		SW:	[yes [yes [(it's been) a long road
19			before you've come th<u>i</u>s far (.) there's been (.) one stay
20			at the <u>shelter</u> there's been <u>two</u> (.) little kids in between
21			.hhh there's a <u>six</u> year stretch (.)
22		C:	[yes
23		SW:	[yes (.) with <u>La</u>sse, (.) different degrees of (.) mental and physical
24	→		violence (.) and (.) <u>now</u> you're (.) in a <u>situation</u> where (.) [you
25		C:	[yes
26	→	SW:	sort of <u>think</u> about and look (.) <u>forward</u> to (.)
27		C:	mm- [m
28	→	SW:	[that.hhhh I can get <u>anything</u> I like at the <u>shop</u> and live
29	→		[(a completely) or[dinary <u>everyday</u>
30		C:	[think- [yes it's <u>exactly</u> these sort of like [ye-e
31	→	SW:	[life (.) in peace and
32	→		quiet.hh[h and er
33		C:	[and it's <u>now</u> that I really realise ho[w <u>important</u> that is
34		SW:	[yes
35		C:	you <u>don't</u> [need anything fancy to [<u>make</u> me hap[py
36		SW:	[yes [ye-es [yep (.)

37		.hhh and still it's only taken, (.) <u>about</u> six weeks I'm [saying that
38	C:	[yes
39	SW:	<u>because</u> it's a fairly <u>short</u> time
40	C:	it [is (.) it is when you <u>think</u> about [:
41	SW:	[.hhhhh [mm-y (.)
42	C:	what a journey it's <u>been</u> so like that was <u>enough</u> of that

At the beginning of the extract, the social worker begins to make her own assessment of the process that the client has gone through, by referring to the client's previous talk: 'what you said . . .' (lines 1–4). The social worker returns to the situation previously described by Lisa, where Lisa's spouse (Lasse) had gained access to the shelter in another town where Lisa had stayed before coming to this shelter. In her talk, the social worker takes the client back to the original scene of events with a very detailed description of the situation (lines 8–10), combining it with the reported speech of the client: 'you thought I'm going to (.) I'm <u>going</u> to die here like this is the last moment of my <u>life</u>' (lines 10, 12 and 14). The social worker quotes the client's voice directly ('I'm <u>going</u> to die . . .', line 12) when describing the horror experienced by the client at that moment. In her next turn, the social worker defines that moment as the worst point in the journey taken by the client (line 15). The social worker's talk begins to take on the structure of a narrative in which the client has travelled a long road before getting to the worst point of the story. The <u>r</u>oad has included many kinds of violence, the births of the children and a stay at a shelter. The client is not a passive recipient of the narrative but participates actively in the discussion by giving feedback that reinforces the social worker's narrative and assessment (lines 11, 13, 16–17 and 22).

However, making an assessment of what was the worst point in the client's life is not the main objective of the social worker's talk; rather, this construction acts in her talk as a yardstick against which the social worker next measures Lisa's current situation. When describing this situation, which is shown in a positive framework, the social worker again uses the direct reported speech of the client: 'I can get <u>anything</u> I like at the <u>shop</u> and live (a completely) ordinary everyday life (.) in peace and quiet' (lines 28–29 and 31–32). The client participates by confirming the social worker's description (lines 25, 27 and 30), until she takes the floor and confirms and completes the description in her own words: 'and it's <u>now</u> that I really realise <u>how</u> <u>important</u> that is' (line 33) and continues: 'you <u>don't</u> need anything fancy to <u>make</u> me happy' (line 35). The social worker, in turn, assumes the position of a listener, providing positive feedback (line 36).

As is demonstrated above, instead of merely reporting the original speech, reported speech fulfils many tasks in the current interaction. The original speech is recontextualised and the speaker uses it in a new context to fulfil certain functions. This example shows all four functions of reported speech. Authenticity and evidence are produced by a detailed description linked to the original situation. In addition, assessment takes place and, among other things, a positive evaluation of the client's situation changing for the better is made. The process of assessment is constructed as a narrative, in which the social worker uses the direct reported speech and thoughts of the client at several points. In the narrative the social worker positions the client again at the worst point in her life, and describes the client's fearful thoughts at that moment using the client's voice, after which she positions the client in the current moment, again with a direct description of the client's current (hopeful) thoughts about her future. The social worker constructs different agencies and identity categories for the client. At the worst point, the identity of a passive agent or even of a potential victim is constructed for the client, whose counterpart is a strong active agent (the husband). The current, altered identity is constructed in considerably different ways: now the client herself is an active agent who can plan an ordinary life, enjoying everyday things in peace and quiet. The client also clearly assumes these definitions as her own, not only by providing agreeing responses at several points, but also by summarising the narrative constructed by the social worker: 'what a journey it's <u>been</u> so like that was <u>enough</u> of that' (line 42) and thus further strengthening her own active agency.

From the viewpoint of social work, reported speech is used in this extract strongly as a tool for change work. It serves as a tool of identity construction in creating a stronger agency for the client, which enables her to detach herself from the violent intimate relationship and to construct a new life. In terms of the interaction this actually succeeds: the conversation is conducted with good, mutual understanding and it becomes shared by the two parties.

Implications for social work practice

In this chapter we have described various functions of reported speech – producing evidence, categorisation, assessment and narrative making – and have demonstrated the use of them in social work interaction. Nearly all social work talk and conversations contain reported speech, although we seldom pay special attention to it. The ways in which reported speech is accomplished in interaction are often firmly connected to the institutional tasks and goals of conversations, as in our two cases where there were the tasks of helping and supporting people suffering from mental health problems or domestic violence. Evidence production and assessment via reported speech can give justifications for professional intervention into suffering, such as the continuation of giving strong mental health support to Julia. Or, when having the functions of categorisation and narrative making, reported speech can be in service of estimating whether the (candidate) clients' needs and problems are such that the social work institution in question can start or continue working with them. For example, by reporting Lisa's own previous talk and ideas, the social worker simultaneously created an identity and narrative for her that the shelter, specialising in serious domestic violence, perhaps no longer has much to offer her.

To conclude, reported speech is not 'just talk', but quoting professionals', clients' and other stakeholders' prior talk influences social work processes and interventions and has consequences for clients' lives – as our two examples clearly showed. In Julia's case the professionals' way of using her prior voice and reported conversations between Julia and themselves portrayed Julia as being at a certain phase of her mental health recovery process. She was assessed as having made some progress but was still seen as needing professional support and control. Lisa's situation was different, however. She was defined as being at the end of both change and client processes and ready to continue her life without the problem of violence. This interpretation of successfully being at the end of clienthood was created strongly by using the client's own reported speech and thoughts from the different phases of the change process.

Producing evidence, categorisation, assessment and narrative making are in many ways at the core of professional social work practices and are also much discussed themes in social work literature. Although these four themes cannot, of course, be reduced to reported speech only, examining closely the interactional usages of reported speech offers relevant viewpoints on them.

Social workers make interventions in people's lives. What they intervene in is linked to the institutional contexts and tasks they are involved with. They are expected to make justified and legitimate interventions and decisions. What has been especially demanded during the last decades is that they need to base their work on proper empirical evidence. This includes making reliable assessments and diagnoses of problems (categorisations) in order to create successful change processes (narratives). In this so-called evidence-based approach, facts are understood as something that can be collected, counted and reported. Hence, they are not seen as being tied to interactional processes. This kind of approach easily ignores everyday fact-producing, assessment and categorisation processes, where reported speech can play a crucial role. The prior talk of clients or other authoritative stakeholders is often presented as empirical evidence when legitimating certain interventions or decisions. But since reported speech is never the same in a reporting context as it was in the original context, it should not be treated as 'pure fact'. For instance, social workers can use doctors' authoritative voices in case conferences to legitimise stronger (or weaker) interventions into the lives of clients, or in accounting for those interventions afterwards. This is neither good nor bad practice but simply unavoidable in social work case talk and thus needs to be made visible and reflected upon.

Who is reporting, whose speech is reported and for what purposes are also issues of power. Professionals need to be explicitly aware that they tend to quote clients' talk in various institutional settings and that this quoting is never 'just' quoting. Hall *et al.* (1999: 565) write that 'one of the tacit assumptions underlying social work is that workers not only act in the best interests of the client but also hear the client'. Reporting clients' speech can be interpreted as evidence of this hearing and can thus be regarded as a sign of ethical practice and client-centredness. It can well be like this, meaning for instance that clients' reported speech is treated as authoritative and with respect in different social work conversations. But clients' prior speech can also be used to blame clients or their voices can be proved wrong by quoting more authoritative voices. Also, an interesting question is how social workers hear and respond to the reported speech presented by clients in professional–client conversations.

Without reported speech social work could not be realised as a change-oriented or process-oriented profession. Remembering and explaining past events at the beginning of clienthood, reasoning and understanding regressions and progresses during clienthood, and orientation to the future necessitate the prior talk of clients and significant others (professionals, relatives, friends etc.) as resources. How these resources are talked into being, both by clients and by professionals in social work interaction, and what the consequences are is a matter of importance. Remembering prior talk can disturb the professional–client relationship, if the memories of the previous talk and discussions are used in a negative framework or if the past talk makes people feel stuck in certain, unchangeable identities ('you have used that same excuse many times before in our meetings and I don't believe you'll ever change'). Alternatively, it can help to create a good relationship with a shared past and task ('do you remember when we first met and you said that I will never recover from this, and look where we are now').

11

DISCOURSE ANALYSIS OF 'ORDINARY' SOCIAL WORK

Christopher Hall, Kirsi Juhila, Maureen Matarese and Carolus van Nijnatten

Social work is interaction

This book has introduced various key discursive and professional concepts to explore social work interaction. The intention of the authors has been to clarify these concepts in the context of data from daily social work practice. How prosaic these data extracts may be, the very ordinary nature of them makes these data, in our view, highly significant. The extracts presented in this book are the daily business of social work. More than that, they represent the heart of social work process. We hope we have shown that even the most ordinary extracts display the critical tension of social work.

The concepts presented in this book have generally been treated individually, each chapter exploring one, although connections between these approaches are also discussed. For example: what does and does not come within the social worker's compass of responsibility may be part of both boundary work and delicate negotiation, or categorisation may arouse client's resistance. While these concepts can be explored on their own, they often co-occur or overlap as the talk develops.

To demonstrate the overlapping of the concepts we present one more illustration from the workplace of social work. Again a demonstration of the richness of what happens in social work communication and the sophisticated conversational strategies of social workers and their clients, the following conversation comes from discussion between a shelter case-worker and her homeless client. They have met several times before, and the client's cousin has been perceived (by the case manager, CM) as a negative influence on the client (C). She begins the meeting by asking her client if he has seen his cousin lately. The ensuing discussion illustrates the convergence of many of the features we have addressed across the chapters in this book, thus emphasising how accountability, narrative, reported speech and so on often occur together within the same stretch of social work talk:

```
1   C:    I just let 'em go. I'm not even dealing with him no more. Just let 'em let
2         'em let 'em do what he wants to do.
3   CM:   right.
4   C:    I'm going to worry about myself from now on. [Forget it.
5   CM:                                                [Good job, let's deal with
6         that first.
7   C:    And I told my sister. I say, You don't have to be here or tell him to come
8         home. You know what I'm saying?(.) He don't come home, I told her I'm
9         not going to be responsible for him over there, I can't. I told her yesterday,
10        I said. I tell 'em I ask ask him nicely to do thins the right way, he don't
11        wanna do it. Let him do what he wants to do.
12  CM:   He's in an adult. You're an adult. And like I told you before y'all going
13        through the same predicament so y'all have to do for yourself. When you
14        get yourself better and you want to help your cousin then that's one thing.
15  C:    Yeah but you see, we're not really in the same predicament because I
16        wanna do something with my self. He doesn't. So.
17  CM:   Well. He has to learn that on his own.
```

In the above extract, we can see narrative: the client's story (lines 7–11) and the caseworker's evaluation of that story (lines 12–14). The client accomplishes categorisation by presenting himself as a 'good' client (lines 4 and 15–16). Accountability provides an excuse for the client's attitude at the shelter, which he attributes to the influence of another client, referred to as 'him' (lines 1–2). Delicacy is displayed, when the caseworker acknowledges that her client is an adult, recognising the uncomfortable position of an adult telling another adult how to live their life while this is often only seen appropriate in adult–child contexts or social worker/doctor–client relationships (line 12). The caseworker even uses reported speech to refer to a previous meeting in which the caseworker provided advice about how her client should act (lines 12 and 13).

Social work is not only inherently about communication, but interactional features, while converging and working together, also make social work possible. This book focused on the daily communicative practices of social workers; it may be seen as a celebration of the central role of social interaction in the social work profession. The book has made visible the complexity of social work practice: how problems become manifest in clients' stories (raised by the social worker), how life perspectives are negotiated and how professionalism is put into practice. This book is about how social work is talked into being.

In various chapters of this book, we tried to include most of the professional actions of social workers. These involve verbal and non-verbal communication – with their clients, their colleagues and their managers in various settings (one-on-one meetings, administrative/staff meetings, case conferences, home visits etc.). These are part and parcel of the talk that constitutes *doing* social work. The cases presented in this volume come from across Europe and the United States and across institutional contexts, including homeless shelters, job centres, centres for children, home visits and social welfare agencies.

Given that so much of social work is achieved through talk and text and given that the field of social work emphasises communication in their instruction (e.g. the development of rapport), it is surprising that the linguistic qualities of social work have received so little empirical attention until recently. Often what we know about social work is hearsay, from reflections that social workers give of their work or by what clients show in satisfaction surveys. This book has worked to highlight what actually happens in day-to-day social work, through a careful, empirical analysis of the features of the talk in that institutional context. Thus, social work becomes a process of interaction between institutional representatives and citizens and a visible and possible object of critical consideration. This book tried to open the black box of social work by analysing its qualities displayed in audio- or video-recordings of actual social work interactions. By recording these interactions it became possible to reflect on what happened in the consulting room or at the home visit.

From measurable interventions to basic social work processes

In the 1980s and 1990s, social work was increasingly criticised for not having appropriate or standardised outcome measures. Without outcome measures, it was difficult to measure productivity, and thus people thought social workers were less successful. As such, beginning in the subfield of child welfare, outcome measures were developed and instituted in order to accelerate productivity. Since the 1980s, new managerialist approaches have been increasingly integrated into social and human service institutions such as schools and social services, and, with a neoliberal philosophical approach, they create social institutions that resemble business institutions in their structure and organisation. New managerialism utilises bureaucratic, management-oriented organisational structures to improve the functioning and efficiency of social institutions. Managers were, therefore, appointed to structure and control professional performance. The positive effects of this were that external evaluation of social work became possible.

Kirkpatrick (2006) suggests that the increased administrative oversight elucidates the processes involved in social work, which is useful for both assessment of social work practice and for social work education. Despite his description of positive attributes, his review of new managerialism is overwhelmingly critical, suggesting that practitioners were not properly trained to deal with the new approach, which was forced on them from the top down. He suggests that 'historically these services were dependent on a sense of professional vocation and a willingness to work "beyond contract". The risk today is that the management reforms are undermining this ethos' (Kirkpatrick 2006: 8). There is also a danger that these assessments are done on the basis of formal features that are easily made observable at the cost of what is more difficult to define precisely in the social work process (van Nijnatten 2010). This presents a disincentive for attending to these unassessed practices in social work. As such, some will simply not engage in those practices because they are not assessed. Others will engage in them anyway even though those practices are advocated but not made relevant by the assessing institution. Harlow (2003) suggests that this approach favours adherence to procedures, guidelines and checklists, which she characterises as 'conveyer belt care' (p. 35), wherein speedy work is applauded and closed cases constitute 'success'. It also leads to 'perverse incentives' where the staff are encouraged to achieve good scores but at the expense of skilled social work (Broadhurst *et al.* 2010; Clarkson 2010). Another negative effect of this institutional reform has been the fragmentation of social work into separate and sometimes arbitrary functional elements, for example the development of call centres as the first contact for social services (Coleman and Harris 2008). Often this is done for reasons of outsourcing and frequently results in deprofessionalisation. The negative effect is that the characteristic social work expertise of knowing and helping people in their complex social context and reckoning with their no less complex personal histories is considered to be no longer necessary. Nothing is further from the truth!

It is obvious that evaluations of social work have to include an assessment of the effects of its interventions on the well-being of clients and the production of social order. Yet it is problematic that social work practices are replaced more and more by informational practices, and that social workers are concerned with finding out what clients *did* rather than trying to understand the rationales of their actions (Parton 2009). Management tools such as time schedules and assessment forms, systems of political organisation (local or national) and systems of professional organisation determine the conversational conditions. They can disrupt social work practice by preventing social workers from making their own narratives (White *et al.* 2009).

In this book, it is demonstrated that social work is more than a collection of interventions whose features may be established more or less objectively and separate from the context in which they are performed. Social work is more than a 'taylorised product' that may be deconstructed in basic elements that then may be reconstructed in an ingenious way to achieve maximum effect. Social work, as is demonstrated in the analyses in this book, is a human enterprise that is based on negotiating meanings (categories, accounts, boundaries) rather than fixed roles and interventions. A sound evaluation of social work has to reckon with both the nature of the problems and the social work (interactional) process.

It seems strange that social work interaction only became an object of serious study in recent years, given the field's emphasis on communication. All the more, it is necessary to present arguments to return to the basic processes of social work and to study social work empirically with the help of recordings of actual social work performances. In this book, social work as a process of interaction between institutional representatives and citizens has become visible and a possible object of critical consideration. To study social work conversation is honouring the social work profession by paying attention to one of its central elements. Although this book contains critical comments on social work practice, it is in the first place an acknowledgement of the complexity of the profession and an appreciation of the relevant work that is done by social workers. We think that evaluation of social work may best be done when interactional processes in the conversations and the institutional context of social work agencies are included. Interactional study gives us the possibility to analyse social work in a theoretically sound way and provides us with a unique and relevant base of evidence.

While social work communication has not so often been the object of empirical study, social work interactions have still been recorded. Many social work conversations were recorded in the frame of video-based interventions (video home training), social work education (learning how to carry on a conversation), performance measurement and implementation integrity (Perepletchikova *et al.* 2007). It is revealing that all these recordings were hardly used to learn more about the dynamics of conversation itself. The analyses in this book were based on interactions that were specifically recorded for the purpose of scientific analysis. We hope that the publication of this book will stimulate social workers and social work agencies to intensify the interactional study of social work: in the first place, by recording themselves, for example conversations with clients, case conferences or interprofessional consultations; and, in the second place, by presenting already recorded conversations for scientific study.

Contribution to social work practice

Interactional phenomena in social work cannot just be approached as elements of professional client interactions, but should always be considered as part of institutional practices. Social workers are not 'nowhere men' and social work is not performed in a social vacuum. It rather takes a crucial position in social policy as a practice connecting governmental initiatives and the private lives of citizens and families. Social work plays a central role in managing social problems, which is a double function of producing social order by helping individuals to get and conserve a decent existence. Social work is at the intersection of autonomy and control, supporting people to live orderly lives and controlling them when they put that order at risk. So social work is challenged both by the individual needs of clients and by governmental directions and budgets (Hjörne *et al.* 2010). Macro-social functions of social work appear at the micro level of conversations between social workers and clients and, the other way around, the course of events in social work conversations has consequences for societal relations. A good conversation with a client depends both on local factors in the dynamics of the conversation itself and on the social conditions of the work.

The chapters in this book go into several interactional aspects of social work. Readers who are familiar with social work will recognise these as elements that almost naturally belong to social work. Where there are attempts to realise changes, there is advice given, resistance offered, accounts made, categories used and boundaries explored. Most of these elements are present in any social work conversation, but for educational reasons we decided to address them in this book in separate chapters.

The key themes from the substantive chapters will be discussed in terms of the potential contribution of discourse analysis to social work. There are three aspects to this discussion. First, a discursive orientation concentrates on what actually happens in practice and therefore questions approaches that formulate social work as either a bureaucratic enterprise that merely implements policy or a practice that operationalises professional mandates. While both may influence what gets done, a discursive approach requires attention to how they are attended to within the complexities of everyday talk and interaction when professionals and clients meet. For example, examining a social worker encounter with a man who is suspected of having committed incest is not just establishing facts about what happened in the family but involves co-constructing a narrative about how things that happened in the past formulates a perspective on the future (van Nijnatten 2007b). Such an orientation points to a more nuanced view of what constitutes social work.

Second, applied conversation and discourse analysis has begun to examine how research findings can set up dialogues with professionals (Willig 1999; Antaki 2011). Current publications on communication in social work rarely examine instances of actual practice or impose an evaluation that comes from outside the data. Discourse-based research may enable professionals to examine their own practice, and have an impact on training and staff development. Many of the authors of this book are engaged in productive researcher/social worker collaborations, sometimes with a research project and a staff development project intertwined (Slembrouck and Hall 2011). At the basis of transcripts of professional–client conversations and video-stimulated recall, interviews, focus groups and discussions were organised (Juhila and Pösö 1999; Hall *et al.* 2010; van Nijnatten and van Doorn 2013). The outcomes of these cooperations may lead immediately to changes in professional practice, but the usefulness of the findings of the discourse analysis is also open to the scrutiny of the professionals. There is considerable interest in reflexive supervision in social work, sometimes supported by government (Social Work Task Force 2009). We suggest that examining instances of actual practice can form a particularly appropriate method for such a practice.

Third, discourse approaches to social work encourage an examination of social work as a mundane practice that is concerned with managing everyday interactional dilemmas, for example offering advice or handling potential disagreement. However, on occasion, issues are addressed that are far from mundane. Social workers confront parents about their care of their children or recommend that vulnerable clients enter residential care. In these instances, managing resistance or seeking agreements require highly complex and sensitive practice. What can discourse analysis offer that can help us understand better such highly charged situations? The analysis of discourse may help to reveal the active elements in daily social work practices that seem self-evident, but in fact have been the essence of professional work over many years. It may also help to disclose professional expertise, which up until now has been taken for granted, in particular regarding social workers' skills to get conversations going, to deal with clients' resistance and to help clients to find their own way. Discourse analysis of social work is an exciting exploratory expedition into the heart of the profession. All the more reason to express the hope that the recording and analysis of interactions in social work practice become part of the routine for staff supervision, professional training and the wider development of social work practice.

Future research

It is natural that interactional analysis of social work has its limitations, especially when it is the only investigatory strategy that has been used. Studies become stronger when they refer to more than one source. So analysis of video-taped interactional sequences may be supplemented with interviews of the people involved (asking them to reflect on the interactions), structured observations and ethnographic approaches. Many interactional studies and analyses are based on small samples, which means that conversational processes that were described cannot just be generalised, because it was not always clear whether the conversations were representative for the populations of social workers and clients. An additional problem is that, in many studies, 'difficult cases' could not be included, because clients or social workers did not want to participate. Sometimes, cases are selected from a bigger data set because relevant processes become visible, but this of course also leads to a selection bias. Future research has to focus on the problem of generalisability of outcomes of interactional analysis of social work conversations. It may point at patterns in social work practice. Yet a different view on this is also possible. Ferguson (2003: 1009) showed in his perspective of 'critical best practice' that case studies are especially suitable for making progress in social work practice, because they identify best practices and professional skills while recognising 'issues of power, inequalities and constraint'.

The authors of this book do not claim to present a systematic outlook of social work, but present some perspectives and instruments that may help to analyse interactional practices that are at the basis of the social work profession. The authors felt privileged to have received permission to take a look behind the scenes of social work. They were impressed by the high quality of social work practice. They hope that this book will contribute to a further exploration of the qualities of social work that show in its daily professional interactions.

APPENDIX

Transcription symbols

The transcription symbols employed in some of the chapters of this book are derived from the system developed by Gail Jefferson (see Atkinson and Heritage 1984: ix–xvi). The authors of the chapters are following these symbols flexibly. Depending on the topic and analytical focus of each chapter, the detail of transcription varies and, following that, the number of symbols used in data extracts. There are also extracts in which periods, commas and questions marks are used in a literary way to make the extracts more readable.

Symbol	Explanation
[	A square bracket marks the start of overlapping speech
↑↓	Upward and downward pointing arrows indicate marked rising and falling shifts in intonation
Underlining	Underlining signals emphasis
CAPITALS	Capital letters indicate a loud voice
°soft°	Raised circles indicate obviously quieter speech
>fast< and <slow>	'Lesser than' and 'greater than' signs indicate talk that is noticeably faster and slower
hhh	Out-breaths
.hhh	In-breaths
ye::s	Colons show degrees of elongation of the prior sound
=	Equals signs indicate no gap between utterances
(1.5)	Numbers in round brackets measure pauses in seconds
(.)	An untimed pause (just hearable)
yes,	A comma marks a continuing intonation
yes.	A full point indicates a stopping fall in tone
yes?	A question mark indicates a rising intonation

( )	Empty parentheses indicate the transcriber's inability to hear what was said
(word)	Parenthesised words are possible hearings
becau-	A hyphen marks a cut-off of the preceding sound
((laugh))	Double brackets indicate an additional comment from the transcriber

(Adapted from Atkinson, J.M. and Heritage, J.C. (eds) (1984) *Structures of Social Action: Studies in conversation analysis*, Cambridge: Cambridge University Press.)

REFERENCES

Abbott, A. (1995) 'Boundaries of social work or social work of boundaries?', *Social Service Review*, 69(4): 545–562.

Adams, R., Dominelli, L. and Payne, M. (eds) (2002) *Critical Practice in Social Work*, Basingstoke: Palgrave.

Allen, D. (2000) 'Doing occupational demarcation: the "boundary-work" of nurse managers in a district general hospital', *Journal of Contemporary Ethnography*, 29(3): 326–356.

Antaki, C. (1994) *Explaining and Arguing: The social organization of accounts*, London: Sage.

Antaki, C. (2008) 'Formulations in psychotherapy', in A. Peräkylä, C. Antaki, S. Vehviläinen and I. Leudar (eds) *Conversation Analysis and Psychotherapy* (pp. 26–42), Cambridge: Cambridge University Press.

Antaki, C. (2011) 'Six kinds of applied conversation analysis', in C. Antaki (ed.) *Applied Conversation Analysis: Intervention and change in institutional talk* (pp. 1–14), Basingstoke: Palgrave Macmillan.

Antaki, C. and Widdicombe, S. (eds) (1998) *Identities in Talk*, London: Sage.

Atkinson, P. (1995) *Medical Talk and Medical Work*, London: Sage.

Atkinson, P. (1997) 'Narrative turn or blind alley?', *Qualitative Health Research*, 7(3): 325–344.

Austin, J.L. (1962) *How to Do Things with Words*, Oxford: Oxford University Press.

Ayre, P. (2001) 'Child protection and the media: lessons from the last three decades', *British Journal of Social Work*, 31(6): 887–901.

Baker, C. (1997) 'Ticketing rules: categorization and moral ordering in a school staff meeting', in S. Hester and P. Eglin (eds) *Culture in Action: Studies in membership categorization analysis* (pp. 77–98), Lanham, MD: International Institute for Ethnomethodology and University Press of America.

Bakhtin, M.M. (1981) *The Dialogic Imagination*, Austin, TX: University of Texas Press.

Baldock, J. and Prior, D. (1981) 'Social workers talking to clients: a study in verbal behaviour', *British Journal of Social Work*, 11(1): 19–38.

Baldwin, C. (2013) *Narrative Social Work: Theory and application*, Bristol: Policy Press.

Banks, S. (2004) *Ethics, Accountability and the Social Professions*, Basingstoke: Palgrave Macmillan.

Barnes, M. and Prior, D. (eds) (2009) *Subversive Citizens: Power, agency and resistance in public services*, Bristol: The Policy Press.

Bartesaghi, M. (2009) 'Conversation and psychotherapy: how questioning reveals institutional answers', *Discourse Studies*, 11(2): 153–177.

Baynham, M. and Slembrouck, S. (1999) 'Speech representation and institutional discourse', *Text*, 19(4): 439–457.

Bergmann, J. (1992) 'Veiled morality: notes on discretion in psychiatry', in P. Drew and J. Heritage (eds) *Talk at Work* (pp. 137–162), Cambridge: Cambridge University Press.

Broadhurst, K., Wastell, D., White, S., Hall, C., Peckover, S., Thompson, K., Pithouse, A. and Davey, D. (2010) 'Performing initial assessment: identifying the latent conditions for error at the front-door of local authority children's services', *British Journal of Social Work*, 40(2): 352–370.

Broadhurst, K., Holt, K. and Doherty, L. (2012) 'Accomplishing parental engagement in child protection practice? A qualitative analysis of parent-professional interaction in pre-proceedings work under the Public Law Online', *Qualitative Social Work*, 11(5): 517–534.

Brown, P. and Levinson, S. (1978) 'Universals of language usage: politeness phenomena', in E. Goody (ed.) *Questions and Politeness* (pp. 56–234), Cambridge: Cambridge University Press.

Bruner, J. (2004) 'Life as narrative', *Social Research*, 54(1): 691–710.

Butler, C.W., Potter, J., Danby, S., Emmison, M. and Hepburn, A. (2010) 'Advice implicative interrogatives: building "client-centred support" in a children's helpline', *Social Psychology Quarterly*, 73(3): 265–287.

Buttny, R. (1993) *Social Accountability in Communication*, London: Sage.

Buttny, R. (1997) 'Reported talk in talking race on campus', *Human Communication Research*, 23(4): 477–506.

Buttny, R. (1998) 'Putting prior talk into context: reported speech and the reporting context', *Research on Language and Social Interaction*, 31(1): 45–58.

Buttny, R. (2004) *Talking Problems: Studies of discursive construction*, Albany, NY: State University of New York Press.

Buttny, R. and Morris, G.H. (2001) 'Accounting', in W.P. Robinson and H. Giles (eds) *The New Handbook on Language and Social Psychology* (pp. 285–302), New York: John Wiley & Sons.

Buttny, R. and Williams, P.L. (2000) 'Demanding respect: the uses of reported speech in discursive constructions of interracial contact', *Discourse & Society*, 11(1): 109–133.

Carey, M. (2008) 'The quasi-market revolution in the head: ideology, discourse, care management', *Journal of Social Work*, 8(4): 341–362.

Caswell, D. and Schultz, I. (2001) *Folket på gaden – om posefolket og gadepraktikken*, Copenhagen: Gyldendal.

Caswell, D., Andersen, H.L., Høybye-Mortensen, M., Markussen, A.M. and Thuesen, S.L. (2011) *Når kassen smækkes i: Analyser af økonomiske sanktioner overfor kontanthjælpsmodtagere*, Copenhagen: AKF Forlaget.

Caswell, D., Eskelinen, L. and Olesen, S.P. (2013) 'Identity work and client resistance underneath the canopy of active employment policy', *Qualitative Social Work*, 12(1): 8–23.

Clarke, J. (2005) 'New Labour's citizens; activated, empowered, responsibilized, abandoned?', *Critical Social Policy*, 25(4): 447–463.

Clarkson, P. (2010) 'Performance measurement in adult social care: looking backwards and forwards', *British Journal of Social Work*, 40(1): 170–187.

Coates, J. (1983) *The Semantics of the Modal Auxillary*, London: Croom-Helm.

Coleman, N. and Harris, J. (2008) 'Calling social work', *British Journal of Social Work*, 38(3): 580–599.

Cooper, F. (2012) *Professional Boundaries in Social Work and Social Care*, London: Jessica Kingsley Press.

Coulmas, F. (1986) 'Reported speech: some general issues', in F. Coulmas (ed.) *Direct and Indirect Speech* (pp. 1–28), Berlin: Mouton de Gruyter.

Couper-Kuhlen, E. (2007) 'Assessing and accounting', in E. Holt and R. Clift (eds) *Reporting Talk: Reported speech in interaction* (pp. 81–119), Cambridge: Cambridge University Press.

Couture, S. and Sutherland, O. (2006) 'Giving advice on advice-giving: a conversation analysis of Karl Tomm's practice', *Journal of Marital and Family Therapy*, 32(3): 329–344.

Crepeau, E. (2000) 'Reconstructing Gloria: a narrative analysis of team meetings', *Qualitative Health Research*, 10(6): 766–787.

Davies, B. and Harré, R. (1990) 'Positioning: the discursive production of selves', *Journal for the Theory of Social Behaviour*, 20(1): 43–63.

D'Cruz, H. and Jones, M. (2004) *Social Work Research: Ethical and political context*, London: Sage.

Dean, M. (1999) *Governmentality: Power and rule in modern society*, London: Sage.

de Certeau, M. (1984) *Practice of Everyday Life*, Berkeley, CA: University of California Press.

de Fina, A. and Schiffrin, D. (2006) *Discourse and Identity*, Cambridge: Cambridge University Press.

Doel, M., Allmark, P., Conway, P., Cowburn, M., Flynn, M., Nelson, P. and Tod, A. (2010) 'Professional boundaries: crossing a line or entering the shadows?', *British Journal of Social Work*, 40(6): 1866–1889.

Donzelot, J. (1979) *The Policing of Families*, New York: Pantheon.

Drew, P. (1998) 'Complaints about transgressions and misconduct', *Research on Language and Social Interaction*, 31(3/4): 295–325.

Drew, P. and Heritage, J. (1992a) 'Analyzing talk at work: an introduction', in P. Drew and J. Heritage (eds) *Talk at Work: Interaction in institutional settings* (pp. 3–65), Cambridge: Cambridge University Press.

Drew, P. and Heritage, J. (eds) (1992b) *Talk at Work: Interaction in institutional settings*, Cambridge: Cambridge University Press.

Edwards, D. (1991) 'Categories are for talking: on the cognitive and discursive bases of categorization', *Theory & Psychology*, 1(4): 515–542.

Edwards, D. (1997) *Discourse and Cognition*, London: Sage.

Edwards, D. (1998) 'The relevant thing about her: social identity categories in use', in C. Antaki and S. Widdicombe (eds) *Identities in Talk* (pp. 15–33), London: Sage.

Edwards, D. and Potter, J. (1992) *Discursive Psychology*, London: Sage.

Erickson, F. (2004) *Talk and Social Theory*, Cambridge: Polity Press.

Eskelinen, L., Olesen, S.P. and Caswell, D. (2010) 'Client contribution in negotiations on employability – categories revised?', *International Journal of Social Welfare*, 19(3): 330–338.

Ezzy, D. (1998) 'Theorizing narrative identity: symbolic interactionism and hermeneutics', *The Sociological Quarterly*, 39(2): 239–252.

Fairclough, N. (1992) *Discourse and Social Change*, Cambridge: Polity Press.

Fairclough, N. (2000) 'Discourse, social theory, and social research: the discourse of welfare reform', *Journal of Sociolinguistics*, 4(2): 163–195.

Feltham, C. (1995) *What is Counselling?*, London: Sage.

Ferguson, H. (2003) 'Outline of a critical best practice perspective on social work and social care', *British Journal of Social Work*, 33(8): 1005–1024.

Ferguson, I. (2007) 'Increasing user choice or privatizing risk? The antinomies of personalization', *British Journal of Social Work*, 37(3): 387–403.

Firth, A. (ed.) (1995) *The Discourse on Negotiation: Studies of language in the workplace*, Oxford: Pergamon.

Fish, S. (1980) *Is There a Text in this Class? The authority of interpretative communities*, Cambridge, MA: Harvard University Press.

Fitzgerald, R. and Austin, H. (2008) 'Accusation, mitigation and resisting guilt in talk', *The Open Communication Journal*, 2: 93–99.

Foucault, M. (1981) *The History of Sexuality, Volume I: An introduction*, Harmondsworth: Penguin.

Foucault, M. (1986) *Archaelogy of Knowledge*, London: Tavistock.

Fox, K.J. (2001) 'Self-change and resistance in prison', in J.F. Gubrium and J.A. Holstein (eds) *Institutional Selves: Troubled identities in a postmodern world* (pp. 176–192), New York and Oxford: Oxford University Press.

Francis, D. and Hester, S. (2004) *An Invitation to Ethnomethodology*, London: Sage.

Fraser, B. (2009) 'Topic orientation markers', *Journal of Pragmatics*, 41(5): 892–898.

Frost, N., Robinson, M. and Anning, A. (2005) 'Social workers in multidisciplinary teams: issues and dilemmas for professional practice', *Child & Family Social Work*, 10(3): 187–196.

Garfinkel, H. (1967) *Studies in Ethnometholodogy*, Englewood Cliffs, NJ: Prentice Hall.

Gee, J. (1991) 'A linguistic approach to narrative', *Journal of Narrative and Life History*, 1(1): 15–39.

Gergen, K. (1994) *Realities and Relationships: Soundings in social construction*, Cambridge, MA: Harvard University Press.

Gieryn, T. (1983) 'Boundary work and the demarcation of science from non-science: strains and interests in the professional ideologies of scientists', *American Sociological Review*, 48(6): 781–795.

Gillespie, A. and Cornish, F. (2010) 'What can be said? Identity as a constraint on knowledge production', *Papers on Social Representations*, 19(5): 1–13.

Goffman, E. (1955) 'On face work: an analysis of ritual elements in social interaction', *Psychiatry: Journal for the Study of Interpersonal Processes*, 18(3): 213–231.

Goffman, E. (1959) *The Presentation of Self in Everyday Life*, Garden City, NY: Anchor.

Goffman, E. (1961/1991) *Asylums: Essays on the social situation of mental patients and other inmates*, London: Penguin Books.

Goffman, E. (1964/1990) *Stigma: Notes on the management of spoiled identity*, London: Penguin Books.

Goffman, E. (1967) *Interaction Ritual: Essays on face-to-face behavior*, Garden City, NY: Anchor.

Goffman, E. (1974) *Frame Analysis: An essay on the organization of experience*, New York: Harper & Row.

Goffman, E. (1981) *Forms of Talk*, Philadelphia, PA: University of Pennsylvania Press.

Goffman, E. (1983) 'The interaction order', *American Sociological Review*, 48(1): 1–17.

Goodwin, C. and Heritage, J. (1990) 'Conversation analysis', *Annual Review of Anthropology*, 19(2): 283–307.

Gregory, M. (2010) 'Reflection and resistance: probation practice and the ethic of care', *British Journal of Social Work*, 40(7): 2274–2290.

Griffiths, L. (1998) 'Humour as resistance to professional dominance in community mental health teams', *Sociology of Health & Illness*, 20(6): 874–895.

Gross, E. and Stone, G. (1964) 'Embarrassment and the analysis of role requirements', *American Journal of Sociology*, 70(1): 1–15.

Gubrium, J. and Holstein, J. (1998) 'Narrative practice and the coherence of personal stories', *The Sociological Quarterly*, 39(1): 163–187.

Gubrium, J. and Holstein, J. (eds) (2001) *Institutional Selves: Troubled identities in a postmodern world*, New York: Open University Press.

Gubrium, J. and Holstein, J. (2009) *Analyzing Narrative Reality*, London: Sage.

Gubrium, J. and Järvinen, M. (eds) (2013) *Turning Troubles into Problems*, London: Routledge.

Günthner, S. (1997) 'Complaint stories: constructing emotional reciprocity among women', in H. Kotthoff and R. Wodak (eds) *Communicating Gender in Context* (pp. 179–218), Amsterdam: John Benjamins.

Haakana, M. (2001) 'Laughter as a patient's resource: dealing with delicate aspects of medical interaction', *Text*, 21(1/2): 187–219.

Haakana, M. (2007) 'Reported thought in complaint stories', in E. Holt and R. Clift (eds) *Reporting Talk: Reported speech in interaction* (pp. 150–178), Cambridge: Cambridge University Press.

Haakana, M. (2010) 'Laughter and smiling: notes on co-occurences', *Journal of Pragmatics*, 42(6): 1499–1512.

Hacking, I. (1986) 'Making up people', in T.C. Heller, M. Sosna and D. Wellbery (eds) *Reconstructing Individualism: Autonomy, individuality, and the self in Western thought* (pp. 222–236), Stanford, CA: Stanford University Press.

Hall, C. (1997) *Social Work as Narrative: Storytelling and persuasion in professional texts*, Aldershot: Ashgate.

Hall, C. and Slembrouck, S. (2007) 'Professional categorization, risk management and inter-agency communication in public inquiries into disastrous outcomes', *British Journal of Social Work*, 39(2): 280–298.

Hall, C., Sarangi, S. and Slembrouck, S. (1999) 'Speech representation and the categorization of the client in social work discourse', *Text*, 19(4): 539–570.

Hall, C., Juhila, K., Parton, N. and Pösö, T. (eds) (2003) *Constructing Clienthood in Social Work and Human Services: Interaction, identities and practices*, London: Jessica Kingsley.

Hall, C., Slembrouck, S. and Sarangi, S. (2006) *Language Practices in Social Work: Categorisation and accountability in child welfare*, London: Routledge.

Hall, C., Slembrouck, S., Haig, E. and Lee, A. (2010) 'The management of professional and other roles during boundary work in child welfare', *International Journal of Social Welfare*, 19(3): 348–357.

Hall, C., Mäkitalo, Å., Slembrouck, S. and Doherty, P. (2012) 'Pursuing trust in child protection meetings: familiarisation and informality', in C.N. Candlin and J. Crichton (eds) *Discourses of Trust* (pp. 111–127), Basingstoke: Palgrave Macmillan.

Hall, S. (2001) 'Foucault: power, knowledge and discourse', in M. Wetherell, S. Taylor and S.J. Yates (eds) *Discourse Theory and Practice: A reader* (pp. 72–81), London: Sage.

Hanlon, N.T. and Rosenberg, M.W. (1998) 'Not-so-new public management and the denial of geography: Ontario health-care reform in the 1990s', *Environment and Planning C: Government and Policy*, 16(5): 559–572.

Harlow, E. (2003) 'New managerialism, social service departments and social work practice today', *Social Work in Action*, 15(2): 29–44.

Have, P. ten (2007) *Doing Conversation Analysis: A practical guide*, London: Sage.

Heath, C. (1988) 'Embarrassment and interactional organization', in P. Drew and A. Wootton (eds) *Erving Goffman: Exploring the interaction order* (pp. 136–150), Cambridge: Polity Press.

Hepburn, A. and Potter, J. (2011) 'Designing the recipient: managing advice resistance in institutional settings, *Social Psychology Quarterly*, 74(2): 216–241.

Heritage, J. (1984) *Garfinkel and Ethnomethodology*, Cambridge: Polity Press.

Heritage, J. (1997) 'Conversation analysis and institutional talk: analyzing data', in D. Silverman (ed.) *Qualitative Analysis: Issues of theory and method* (pp. 222–245), London: Sage.

Heritage, J. (2001) 'Goffman, Garfinkel and conversation analysis', in M. Wetherell, S. Taylor and S.J. Yates (eds) *Discourse Theory and Practice: A reader* (pp. 47–56), London: Sage.

Heritage, J. and Atkinson, J.M. (1984) 'Introduction', in J.M. Atkinson and J. Heritage (eds) *Structures of Social Action: Studies in conversation analysis* (pp. 1–15), Cambridge: Cambridge University Press.

Heritage, J. and Lindström, A. (2012) 'Advice giving – terminable and interminable: the case of British health visitors', in H. Limberg and M. Locher (eds) *Advice in Discourse*, Amsterdam: John Benjamins Publishing.

Heritage, J. and Maynard, D. (2006) *Communication in Medical Care: Interaction between primary care physicians and patients*, Cambridge: Cambridge University Press.

Heritage, J. and Raymond, S. (2005) 'The terms of agreement: indexing epistemic authority and subordination in talk-in-interaction', *Social Psychology Quarterly*, 68(1): 15–38.

Heritage, J. and Sefi, S. (1992) 'Dilemmas of advice: aspects of the delivery and reception of advice in interactions between health visitors and first time mothers', in P. Drew and J. Heritage (eds) *Talk at Work: Interaction in institutional settings* (pp. 359–417), Cambridge: Cambridge University Press.

Hernes, T. (2004) 'Studying composite boundaries: a framework of analysis', *Human Relations*, 57(1): 9–29.

Hester, S. (1998) 'Membership categories and their practical and institutional relevance', in C. Antaki and S. Widdicombe (eds) *Identities in Talk* (pp. 133–150), London: Sage.

Hester, S. and Eglin, P. (1997) *Culture in Action: Studies in membership categorization analysis 1997*, Lanham, MD: International Institute for Ethnomethodology and University Press of America.

Hitzler, S. (2011) 'Fashioning a proper institutional position: professional identity work in the triadic structure of the care planning conference', *Qualitative Social Work*, 10(3): 293–310.

Hjörne, E. and Mäkitalo, Å. (2008) 'PÅ vems premisser? Institutionell argumentation och socialisering av barn och vuxna', in M. Molin, A. Gustavsson and H.-E. Hermansson (eds) *Meningsskapande och delaktighet: vår tids social-pedagogik* (pp. 187–207), Göteborg: Daidalos.

Hjörne, E. and Säljö, R. (2012) 'Institutional labeling and pupil careers: negotiating identities of children who do not fit in', in T. Cole, H. Daniels and J. Visser (eds) *Routledge International Companion to Emotional and Behavioural Difficulties* (pp. 40–47), London: Routledge.

Hjörne, E., Juhila, K. and van Nijnatten, C. (2010) 'Negotiating dilemmas in the practices of street-level welfare work', *International Journal of Social Welfare*, 19(3): 303–309.

Hollander, J.A. and Einwohner, T.L. (2004) 'Conceptualizing resistance', Sociological Forum, 19(4): 533–554.

Hollis, F. (1964) *Casework: A psychosocial therapy*, New York: Random House.

Holt, E. (1996) 'Reporting on talk: the use of direct reported speech in conversation', *Research on Language and Social Interaction*, 29(3): 219–245.

Holt, E. (2000) 'Reporting and reacting: concurrent responses to reported speech', *Research on Language and Social Interaction*, 33(4): 425–454.

Holt, E. and Clift, R. (eds) (2007) *Reporting Talk: Reported speech in interaction*, Cambridge: Cambridge University Press.

Høybye-Mortensen, M. (2013) '*I velfærdsstatens frontlinje: Administration, metoder og beslutningstagning (At the Frontline of the Welfare State: Administration, methods and decisionmaking)*', Copenhagen: Hans Reitzels Forlag.

Hutchby, I. (2002) 'Resisting the incitement to talk in child counselling: aspects of the utterance "I don't know"', *Discourse Studies*, 4(2): 147–168.

Hutchby, I. and Wooffitt, R. (1998) *Conversation Analysis*, Cambridge: Polity Press.

Hydén, L.-C. (1996) 'Applying for money: the encounter between social workers and clients – a question of morality', *British Journal of Social Work*, 26(6): 843–860.

Hydén, L.-C. (2001) 'Who!? Identity in institutional contexts', in M. Seltzer, C. Kullberg, S.P. Olesen and I. Rostila (eds) *Listening to the Welfare State* (pp. 213–240), Aldershot: Ashgate.

Hyden, M. and Overlien, C. (2005) 'Applying narrative analysis to the process of confirming or disregarding cases of suspected sexual abuse', *Child and Family Social Work*, 10(1): 57–65.

Ijäs-Kallio, T., Ruusuvuori, J. and Peräkylä, A. (2010) 'Patient resistance towards diagnosis in primary care: implications for concordance', *Health*, 14(5): 505–522.

Iser, W. (1974) *The Implied Reader*, Baltimore, MD: Johns Hopkins University Press.

Jayyusi, L. (1984) *Categorization and the Moral Order*, Boston, MA: Routledge & Kegan Paul.

Jayyusi, L. (1991) 'Values and moral judgement: communicative praxis as a moral order', in G. Button (ed.) *Ethnomethodology and the Human Sciences* (pp. 227–251), Cambridge: Cambridge University Press.

Jefferson, G. (1984) 'On the organization of laughter in talk about troubles', in J.M. Atkinson and J. Heritage (eds) *Structures of Social Action: Studies in conversation analysis* (pp. 346–369), Cambridge: Cambridge University Press.

Jefferson, G. (1984) 'Notes on a systematic deployment of the acknowledgement tokens "yeah" and "mm hm"', *Papers in Linguistics*, 17: 197–216.

Jefferson, G. and Lee, J. (1992) 'The rejection of advice: managing the problematic convergence of a trouble-telling and service encounter', in P. Drew and J. Heritage (eds) *Talk at Work: Interaction in institutional settings*, Cambridge: Cambridge University Press.

Jokinen, A., Juhila, K. and Pösö, T. (eds) (1999) *Constructing Social Work Practices*, Aldershot: Ashgate.

Jokinen, A., Juhila, K. and Suoninen, E. (2001) 'Negotiating meanings in and through interactional positions in professional helping work', in M. Seltzer, C. Kullberg, S.P. Olesen and I. Rostila (eds) *Listening to the Welfare State* (pp. 39–54), Aldershot: Ashgate.

Juhila, K. (2003) 'Creating a "bad" client: disalignment of institutional identities in social work interaction', in C. Hall, K. Juhila, N. Parton and T. Pösö (eds) *Constructing Clienthood in Social Work and Human Services* (pp. 83–95), London: Jessica Kingsley.

Juhila, K. (2004) 'Talking back to stigmatised identities: negotiation of culturally dominant categorizations in interviews with shelter residents', *Qualitative Social Work*, 3(3): 259–275.

Juhila, K. and Abrams, L.S. (2011) 'Special issue editorial: constructing identities in social work settings', *Qualitative Social Work*, 10(13): 277–292.

Juhila, K. and Pösö, T. (1999) 'Negotiating constructions: rebridging social work research and practice in the context of probation work', in A. Jokinen, K. Juhila and T. Pösö (eds) *Constructing Social Work Practices* (pp. 274–303), Aldershot: Ashgate.

Juhila, K. and Raitakari, S. (2010) 'Ethics in professional interaction: justifying the limits of helping in a supported housing unit', *Ethics and Social Welfare*, 4(1): 57–71.

Juhila, K., Hall, C. and Raitakari, S. (2010) 'Accounting for the client's troublesome behaviour in a supported housing unit: blames, excuses and responsibility in professionals' talk', *Journal of Social Work*, 10(1): 59–79.

Juhila, K., Hall, C. and Raitakari, S. (in preparation) 'Accepting and negotiating service users' choices in mental health transition meetings'.

Juhila, K., Raitakari, S. and Günther, K. (forthcoming) 'Negotiating mental health rehabilitation plans: joint future talk and clashing time talk in professional client interaction'.

Juhila, K., Saario, S., Günther, K. and Raitakari, S. (2011) 'Reported client–practitioner conversations as assessment in mental health practitioners' meeting talk'. Paper presented at the Eighth DANASWAC seminar, Utrecht, June.

Kadushin, A. and Kadushin, G. (1997) *The Social Work Interview: A guide for human service professionals*, New York: Columbia University Press.

Kirkpatrick, I. (2006) 'Taking stock of the new managerialism in English social services', *Social Work & Society*, 4(1): 14–24.

Komter, M. (2003) 'The interactional dynamics of eliciting a confession in a Dutch police interrogation', *Research on Language and Social Interaction*, 36(4): 433–470.

Kurri, K. (2005) *The Invisible Moral Order: Agency, accountability and responsibility in therapy talk*, Jyväskylä: University of Jyväskylä.

Kurri, K. and Wahlström, J. (2005) 'Placement of responsibility and moral reasoning in couple therapy', *Journal of Family Therapy*, 27(4): 352–369.

Labov, W. (1972) *Language in the Inner City: Studies in the Black English vernacular*, Pittsburgh, PA: University of Pennsylvania Press.

Labov, W. and Waletzky, J. (1967) 'Narrative analysis: oral versions of personal experience', in J. Helms (ed.) *Essays in the Verbal and Visual Arts*, Seattle, WA: University of Washington Press.

Lefebvre, H. (1991) *The Production of Space*, Oxford: Basil Blackwell.

Leppänen, V. (1998) 'The straightforwardness of advice: advice-giving in interactions between Swedish district nurses and patients', *Research in Language and Social Interaction*, 31(2): 209–239.

Leydon, G. (2008) '"Yours is potentially serious but most of these are cured": optimistic communication in UK outpatient oncology consultation', *Psycho-Oncology*, 17(11): 1081–1088.

Linell, P. and Bredmar, M. (1996) 'Reconstructing topical sensitivity: aspects of face-work in talks between midwives and expectant mothers', *Research on Language and Social Interaction*, 29(4): 347–379.

Linell, P. and Fredin, E. (1995) 'Negotiating terms in social welfare office talk', in A. Firth (ed.) *The Discourse of Negotiation.* (pp. 299–318), Oxford: Pergamon Press.

Lipsky, M. (1980) *Street-level Bureaucracy: Dilemmas of the individual in public services*, New York: Russel Sage Foundation.

Locher, M. and Limberg, H. (2012) 'Introduction to Limberg', in H. Limberg and M. Locher (eds) *Advice in Discourse* (pp. 1–27), Amsterdam: John Benjamins Publishing.

McAdams, D. (1996) 'Personality, modernity and the storied self: a contemporary framework for studying persons', *Psychological Inquiry*, 7(4): 295–321.

McDaniels, S. (1995) *Identity Construction through Narrative: The impact of chaotic environments and negative affective experiences of childhood*. Doctoral thesis, University of Chicago. Available at www.icsw.edu/_dissertations/mcdaniels_1995.pdf (no longer available).

Mchoul, A. (1978) 'The organization of turns at formal talk in the classroom', *Language in Society*, 7(2): 183–213.

MacMartin, C. (2008) 'Resisting optimistic questions in narrative and solution-focused therapies', in A. Peräkylä, C. Antaki, S. Vehviläinen and I. Leudar (eds) *Conversation Analysis and Psychotherapy* (pp. 80–99), Cambridge: Cambridge University Press.

Mäkitalo, Å. (2002) *Categorizing Work: Knowing, arguing, and social dilemmas in vocational guidance*, Göteborg: Acta Universitatis Gothoburgensis.

Mäkitalo, Å. (2003) 'Accounting practices as situated knowing: dilemmas and dynamics in institutional categorization', *Discourse Studies*, 5(4): 495–516.

Mäkitalo, Å. (2006) 'Effort on display: unemployment and the interactional manage-ment of moral accountability', *Symbolic Interaction*, 29(4): 531–555.

Mäkitalo, Å. and Säljö, R. (2002a) 'Invisible people: institutional reasoning and reflexivity in the production of services and "social facts" in public employment agencies', *Mind, Culture, and Activity*, 9(3): 160–178.

Mäkitalo, Å. and Säljö, R. (2002b) 'Talk in institutional context and institutional context in talk: categories as situated practices', *TEXT*, 22(1): 57–82.

Maluccio, A. (1979) *Learning from Clients: Interpersonal help as viewed by clients and social workers*, New York: Free Press.

Manthey, T., Knowles, B., Asher, D. and Wahab, A. (2011) 'Strengths-based practice and motivational interviewing', *Advances in Social Work*, 12(2): 126–151.

Margolin, L. (1997) *Under the Cover of Kindness: The invention of social work*, Charlotteville, VA: University of Virginia.

Martin, F. (1998) 'Tales of transition: self-narrative and direct scribing in exploring care-leaving', *Child and Family Social Work*, 3(1): 1–12.

Marvasti, A. (2002) 'Constructing the service-worthy homeless through narrative editing', *Journal of Contemporary Ethnography*, 31(5): 615–651.

Matarese, M. and van Nijnatten, C. (under review) 'Client insistence: rethinking resistance in caseworker-client interaction', *Discourse Processes*.

May-Chahal, C. and Har, M.K. (2011) 'Breaching private life with authority: finding a necessary feature of social work', *Qualitative Social Work*, 10(4): 520–536.

Maynard, D. (1991) 'Interaction and asymmetry in clinical discourse', *American Journal of Sociology*, 97(2): 448–495.

Mead, G. (1935) *Mind, Self and Society*, Chicago, IL: Chicago University Press.

Mehan, H. (1993) 'Beneath the skin and between the ears: a case study in the politics of representation', in J. Lave and S. Chaiklin (eds) *Understanding Practice: Perspectives on activity and context* (pp. 241–268), Cambridge, MA: Cambridge University Press.

Mehan, H., Hertweck, A. and Meihls, J.L. (1986) *Handicapping the Handicapped: Decision making in students' educational careers*, Stanford, CA: Stanford University Press.

Messmer, H. and Hitzler, S. (2011) 'Declientification: undoing client identities in care planning conferences on the termination of residential care', *British Journal of Social Work*, 41(4): 778–798.

Miehls, D. and Moffatt, K. (2000) 'Constructing social work identity based on the reflexive self', *British Journal of Social Work*, 30(3): 339–348.

Miller, G. (1991) *Enforcing the Work Ethic: Rhetoric and everyday life in a work incentive program*, Albany, NY: State University of New York Press.

Miller, G. (2003) 'Writers', clients', counsellors' and readers' perspectives in constructing resistant clients', in C. Hall, K. Juhila, N. Parton and T. Pösö (eds) *Constructing Clienthood in Social Work and Human Services* (pp. 193–207), London: Jessica Kingsley.

Muntigl, P. and Choi, T.C. (2010) 'Not remembering as a practical epistemic resource in couples therapy', *Discourse Studies*, 12(3): 331–356.

Myers, G. (1999) 'Functions of reported speech in group discussions', *Applied Linguistics*, 20(3): 376–401.

Nancarrow, A. and Borthwick, S. (2005) 'Dynamic professional boundaries in the healthcare workforce', *Sociology of Health and Illness*, 27(7): 897–919.

Noordegraaf, M. (2008) *Assessment in Action: Assessing and displaying suitability for adoptive parenthood through text and talk*, Wageningen: Ponsen & Looijen.

Noordegraaf, M., van Nijnatten, C. and Elbers, E. (2008) 'Assessing suitability for adoptive parenthood: hypothetical questions as part of ongoing conversation', *Discourse Studies*, 10(5): 655–672.

Noordegraaf, M., van Nijnatten, C. and Elbers, E. (2009) 'How social workers start to assess the suitability of prospective adoptive parents', *Research on Language and Social Interaction*, 42(3): 276–298.

Norrick, N. and Spitz, A. (2008) 'Humor as a resource for mitigating conflict in interaction', *Journal of Pragmatics*, 40(10): 1661–1686.

Ochs, E. and Capps, L. (2001) *Living Narrative: Creating lives in everyday storytelling*, Cambridge, MA: Harvard University Press.

Olaison, A. (2010) 'Creating images of old people as home care receivers: categorizations of needs in social work case files', *Qualitative Social Work*, 9(4): 500–518.

Olaison, A. and Cedersund, E. (2006) 'Assessments for home care: negotiating solutions for individual needs', *Journal of Aging Studies*, 20(4): 367–388.

O'Leary, P., Tsui, M.-S. and Ruch, G. (2012) 'The boundaries of the social work relationship revisited: towards a connected, inclusive and dynamic conceptualisation', *British Journal of Social Work* (January): 1–19. Available at http://bjsw.oxfordjournals.org/content/early/2012/01/10/bjsw.bcr181.full.pdf+html (accessed 10 January 2012).

Osvaldsson, K. (2004) '"I don't have no damn cultures": doing normality in a "deviant" setting', *Qualitative Research in Psychology*, 1(3): 239–264.

Paoletti, I. (2001) 'Membership categories and time appraisal in interviews with family caregivers of disabled elderly', *Human Studies*, 24(4): 293–325.

Parton, N. (2009) 'Challenges to practice and knowledge in child welfare social work: from the "social" to the "informational"', *Children and Youth Services Review*, 31(7): 715–721.

Parton, N. and O'Byrne, P. (2000) *Constructive Social Work: Towards new theory and practice*, London: Palgrave Macmillan.

Payne, M. (1997) *Modern Social Work Theory*, 2nd edn, London: Macmillan.

Peräkylä, A. (1995) *AIDS Counselling: Institutional interaction and clinical practice*, Cambridge: Cambridge University Press.

Peräkylä, A. (2002) 'Agency and authority: extended responses to diagnostic statements in primary care encounters', *Research on Language and Social Interaction*, 35(2): 219–247.

Peräkylä, A. (2005) *AIDS Counselling: Institutional interaction and clinical practice*, Cambridge: Cambridge University Press.

Peräkylä. A., Antaki C., Vehviläinen, S. and Leudar, I. (eds) (2008a) *Conversation Analysis and Psychotherapy*, Cambridge: Cambridge University Press.

Peräkylä. A., Antaki C., Vehviläinen, S. and Leudar, I. (2008b) 'Analysing psychotherapy in practice', in A. Peräkylä, C. Antaki, S. Vehviläinen and I. Leudar (eds) *Conversation Analysis and Psychotherapy* (pp. 5–25), Cambridge: Cambridge University Press.

Perepletchikova, F., Treat, T. and Kazdin, A. (2007) 'Treatment integrity in psychotherapy research: analysis of the studies and examination of the associated factors', *Journal of Consulting and Clinical Psychology*, 75(6): 829–841.

Pilnick, A. and Coleman, T. (2003) '"I'll give up smoking when you get me better": patients' resistance to attempts to problematise smoking in general practice (GP) consultations', *Social Science and Medicine*, 57(1): 135–145.

Pithouse, A. (1998) *Social Work: The organization of an invisible trade*, Aldershot: Ashgate.

Pithouse, A. and Atkinson, P. (1988) 'Telling the case: occupational narrative in a social work office', in N. Coupland (ed.) *Styles of Discourse* (pp. 183–200), Beckenham: Croom Helm.

Poindexter, C. (2002) 'Meaning from methods: re-presenting narratives of an HIV-affected caregiver', *Qualitative Social Work*, 1(1): 59–78.

Pomerantz, A. (1986) 'Extreme case formulations: a way of legitimizing claims', *Human Studies*, 9(2/3): 219–229.

Potter, J. (1996) *Representing Reality: Discourse, rhetoric and social construction*, London: Sage.

Potter, J. (2012) 'Discourse analysis and discursive psychology', in H. Cooper (ed.) *APA Handbook of Research Methods in Psychology, Volume 2: Research designs: quantitative, qualitative, neuropsychological, and biological* (pp. 111–130), Washington, DC: American Psychological Association Press.

Potter, J. and Wetherell, M. (1987) *Discourse and Social Psychology: Beyond attitudes and behaviour*, London: Sage.

Psathas, G. (1995) *Conversation Analysis: The study of talk-in-interaction*, Qualitative Research Methods Series 35, London: Sage.

Pudlinski, C. (2002) 'Accepting and rejecting advice as competent peers: caller dilemmas on a warm line', *Discourse Studies*, 4(4): 481–500.

Pugh, R. (2007) 'Dual relationships: personal and professional boundaries in rural social work', *British Journal of Social Work*, 37(8): 1405–1423.

Raitakari, S. (2006) *Neuvottelut ja merkinnät minuuksista: Vuorovaikutuksellisuus ja retorisuus lastensuojeluyksikön palavereissa ja tukisuunnitelmissa*, Tampere: Tampere University Press, Acta Universitatis Tamperensis 1183.

Reamer, F. (2003) 'Boundary issues in social work: managing dual relationships', *Social Work*, 48(1): 121–133.

Reid, W. and Shapiro, B. (1969) 'Client reactions to advice', *The Social Services Review*, 43(2): 165–173.

Ricoeur, P. (1985) 'Narrated time', *Philosophy Today*, 29(4): 259–272.

Ricoeur, P. (1988) *Time and Narrative, Volume 3*, Chicago, IL: University of Chicago Press.

Ricoeur, P. (1991) 'Life in quest of narrative', in D. Wood (ed.) *On Paul Ricoeur: Narrative and interpretation* (pp. 20–33), London: Routledge.

Riemann, G. (2005) 'Trying to make sense of cases: features and problems of social workers' case discussions', *Qualitative Social Work*, 4(4): 413–430.

Riessman, C.K. (2000) 'Stigma and everyday resistance practices: childless women in South India', *Gender & Society*, 14(1): 111–135.

Riessman, C.K. (2008) *Narrative Methods for the Human Sciences*, Thousand Oaks, CA: Sage.

Riessman, C.K. and Quinney, L. (2005) 'Narrative in social work', *Qualitative Social Work*, 4(4): 391–412.

Roe, D. and Davidson, L. (2005) 'Self and narrative in schizophrenia: time to author a new story', *Medical Humanities*, 31(2): 89–94.

Roscoe, K., Carson, A. and Madoc-Jones, L. (2011) 'Narrative social work: conversations between theory and practice', *Journal of Social Work Practice*, 25(1): 47–61.

Rose, N. (2002) *Powers of Freedom: Reframing political thought*, Cambridge: Cambridge University Press.

Rutten, K., Mottart, A. and Soetaert, R. (2010) 'Narrative and rhetoric in social work education', *British Journal of Social Work*, 40(2): 480–495.

Ruusuvuori, J. (2005) ' "Empathy" and "sympathy" in action: attending to patients' troubles in Finnish homeopathic and general practice consultations', *Social Psychology Quarterly*, 68(3): 204–222.

Saario, S. (2012) 'Managerial reforms and specialised psychiatric care: a study of resistive practices performed by mental health practitioners', *Sociology of Health and Illness*, 34(6): 896–910.

Saario, S. and Raitakari, S. (2010) 'Contractual audit and mental health rehabilitation: a study of formulating effectiveness in a Finnish supported housing unit', *International Journal of Social Welfare*, 19(3): 321–329.

Sacks, H. (1963/1984) 'On doing "being ordinary" ', in J.M. Atkinson and J. Heritage (eds) *Structures of Social Action: Studies in conversation analysis* (pp. 413–429), London: Macmillan.

Sacks, H. (1972a) On the analyzability of stories by children', in J. Coulter (ed.) *Ethnomethodological Sociology*, pp. 254–270, Aldershot: Edward Elgar.

Sacks, H. (1972b) 'An initial investigation of the usability of conversational data for doing sociology', in D. Sudnow (ed.) *Studies in Social Interaction* (pp. 31–74), Glencoe, IL: Free Press.

Sacks, H. (1992) *Lectures on Conversation* (ed. G. Jefferson), Oxford: Blackwell.

Sacks, H., Schegloff, E.A. and Jefferson, G. (1974) 'A simplest systematics for the organization of turn-taking for conversations', *Language*, 50(4): 696–735.

Sanders, T. and Harrison, S. (2008) 'Professional legitimacy claims in the multi-disciplinary workplace: the case of heart failure care', *Sociology of Health and Illness*, 30(2): 289–308.

Sarangi, S. and Slembrouck, S. (1996) *Language, Bureaucracy and Social Control*, London: Longman.

Schegloff, E.A. (1992) 'On talk and its institutional occasion', in P. Drew and J. Heritage (eds) *Talk at Work: Interaction in institutional settings* (pp. 101–134), Cambridge: Cambridge University Press.

Schegloff, E.A. (2007) *Sequence Organization in Interaction: A primer in conversation analysis*, Cambridge: Cambridge University Press.

Scott, M. and Lyman, S. (1968) 'Accounts', *American Sociological Review*, 33(1): 46–62.

Seltzer, M., Kullberg K., Olesen, S.P. and Rostila, I. (eds) (2001) *Listening to the Welfare State*, Aldershot, Ashgate.

Shotter, J. (1993) *Conversational Realities: Constructing life through language*, London: Sage.

Shuman, A. (2006) 'Entitlement and empathy in personal narrative', *Narrative Inquiry*, 16(1): 148–155.

Silverman, D. (1987) *Communication and Medical Practice: Social relations in the clinic*, London: Sage.

Silverman, D. (1997) *Discourses of Counselling: HIV counselling as social interaction*, London: Sage.

Silverman, D. (1998) *Harvey Sacks: Social science and conversation analysis*, New York: Oxford University Press.

Silverman, D. (2000) 'Routine pleasure: the aesthetics of the mundane', in S. Linstead and H. Hopfi (eds) *The Aesthetics of Organisation*, London: Sage.

Silverman, D. (2007) *A Very Short, Fairly Interesting and Reasonably Cheap Book about Qualitative Research*, London: Sage.

Silverman, D. (2011) *Interpreting Qualitative Data*, 4th edn, London: Sage.

Silverman, D. and Peräkylä, A. (1990) 'AIDS counselling: the interactional organization of talk about "delicate" issues', *Sociology of Health and Illness*, 12(3): 293–318.

Slembrouck, S. and Hall, C. (2003) 'Caring but not coping: fashioning a legitimate parent identity', in C. Hall, K. Juhila, N. Parton and T. Pösö (eds) *Constructing Clienthood in Social Work and Human Services* (pp. 44–61), London: Jessica Kingsley.

Slembrouck, S. and Hall, C. (2011) 'Family support and home visiting: understanding communication, "good practice" and interactional skills', in C. Candlin and S. Sarangi (eds) *Handbook of Applied Linguistics: Communication in the professions* (pp. 481–497), Berlin: Mouton de Gruyter.

Smith, D. (1978) ' "K is mentally ill": the anatomy of a factual account', *Sociology*, 12(1): 23–53.

Smith, D. (1993) *Texts, Facts and Femininity: Exploring the relations of ruling*, London: Routledge.

Social Work Task Force (2009) *Building a Safe, Confident Future: The final report of the Social Work Task Force*, London: Department for Children, Schools and Families.

Solberg, J. (2011) 'Activation encounters: dilemmas of accountability in constructing clients' as "knowledgeable"', *Qualitative Social Work*, 10(3): 381–398.

Speer, S. and Parsons, C. (2006) 'Gatekeeping gender: some features of the use of hypothetical questions in the psychiatric assessment of transsexual patients', *Discourse & Society*, 17(6): 785–812.

Stivers, T. (2005) 'Parent resistance to physicians' treatment recommendations: one resource for initiating a negotiation of the treatment decision', *Health Communication*, 18(1): 41–47.

Stivers, T. (2008) 'Stance, alignment and affiliation during storytelling: when nodding is a token of affiliation', *Research on Language and Social Interaction*, 41(1): 31–57.

Stokoe, E. (2009) 'Doing actions with identity categories: complaints and denials in neighbour disputes', *Talk and Text*, 29(1): 75–97.

Stokoe, E. and Edwards, D. (2006) 'Story formulations in talk-in-interaction', *Narrative Inquiry*, 16(1): 56–65.

Stokoe, E. and Edwards, D. (2007) ' "Black this, black that": racial insults and reported speech in neighbour complaints and police interrogations', *Discourse & Society*, 18(3): 337–372.

Striker, P. (1990) 'Social work and self-determination', *British Journal of Social Work*, 20(3): 221–236.

Suoninen, E. (1999) 'Doing delicacy in institutions of helping: a case of probation office interaction', in A. Jokinen, K. Juhila and T. Pösö (eds) *Constructing Social Work Practices* (pp. 103–115), Aldershot: Ashgate.

Suoninen, E. and Jokinen, A. (2005) 'Persuasion in social work interviewing', *Qualitative Social Work*, 4(4): 469–487.

Suoninen, E. and Wahlström, J. (2009) 'Interactional positions and the production of identities: negotiating fatherhood in family therapy', *Communication and Medicine*, 6(2): 199–209.

Tannen, D. (2007) *Talking Voices: Repetition, dialogue and imagery in conversational discourse*, 2nd edn, Cambridge: Cambridge University Press.

Tannen, D. and Wallat, C. (1987) 'Interactive frames and knowledge schemas in interaction: examples from a medical interview', *Social Psychology Quarterly*, 50(2): 205–216.

Taylor, C. and White, S. (2000) *Practising Reflexivity in Health and Welfare: Making knowledge*, Buckingham: Open University Press.

Taylor, P. (2003) 'Humbolt's rift: managerialism in education and complicit intellectuals', *European Political Science*, 3(1): 1–7.

Taylor, S. and Wetherell, M. (eds) (2001) *Discourse as Data: A guide for analysis*, London: Sage.

Themessl-Huber, M., Humphris, G., Dowell, J., Macgillivray, S., Rushmer, R. and Williams, B. (2008) 'Audio-visual recording of patient–GP consultations for research purposes: a literature review on recruiting rates and strategies', *Patient Education and Counselling*, 71(2): 157–168.

Thomas, R. and Davies, A. (2005) 'Theorizing the micropolitics of resistance: new public management and managerial identities in the UK public services', *Organisation Studies*, 26(5): 683–706.

Tilly, C. (2004) 'Social boundary mechanisms', *Philosophy of the Social Sciences*, 34(2): 211–236.

Trevithick, P., Richards, S., Ruch, G., Moss, B., Lines, L. and Manor, O. (2004) *SCIE Knowledge Review 6: Teaching and learning communication skills in social work education*, London: Social Care Institute for Excellence.

Urek, M. (2005) 'Making a case in social work: the construction of an unsuitable mother', *Qualitative Social Work*, 4(4): 451–467.

Usita, P., Hyman, I. and Herman, K. (1998) 'Narrative intentions: listening to life stories in Alzheimer's disease', *Journal of Aging Studies*, 12(2): 185–197.

Välimaa, O. (2011) *Kategoriat ongelman selontekoina: pitkäaikaistyöttömyydestä neuvotteleminen ja sen rakentuminen haastattelupuheessa*, Tampere: Tampere University Press, Acta Universitatis Tamperensis 1589.

van Nijnatten, C. (2005) 'The presentation of authority in encounters with mandated clients', *Advances in Sociology Research*, 2: 57–79.

van Nijnatten, C. (2007a) 'The discourse of empowerment: a dialogical self theoretical perspective on the interface of person and institution in social service settings', *International Journal of Dialogical Science*, 2(1): 337–359.

van Nijnatten, C. (2007b) 'Balancing care and control: good practice in assessing an allegation of child sexual abuse', *Social Work and Social Sciences Review*, 12(3): 29–47.

van Nijnatten, C. (2010) *Children's Agency, Children's Welfare: A dialogical approach to child development, policy and practice*, Bristol: Policy Press.

van Nijnatten, C. (2013) 'Downgrading as a counterstrategy: a case study in child welfare', *Child & Family Social Work*, 18(2): 139–148.

van Nijnatten, C. and Hofstede, G. (2003) 'Parental identity under construction: discourse and conversation analysis of a family supervision order', in K. Juhila, T. Pösö, C. Hall and N. Parton (eds) *Constructing Clienthood in Social Work and Human Services: Interaction, identities, and practices* (pp. 96–111), London: Jessica Kingsley.

van Nijnatten, C. and van Doorn, F. (2013) 'The role of play activities in facilitating child participation in psychotherapy', *Discourse Studies*, 15(5): forthcoming.

van Nijnatten, C., Hoogsteder, M. and Suurmond, J. (2001) 'Communication in care and coercion: institutional interactions between family supervisors and parents', *British Journal of Social Work*, 31(5): 705–720.

Vehviläinen, S. (1999) *Structures of Counselling Interaction: A conversation analytic study of counselling encounters in career guidance training*, Helsinki: Helsinki University Press.

Vehviläinen, S. (2001) 'Evaluative advice in educational counselling: the use of disagreement in the "stepwise entry" to advice', *Research on Language and Social Interaction*, 34(3): 371–398.

Vehviläinen, S. (2008) 'Identifying and managing resistance in psychoanalytic interaction', in A. Peräkylä, C. Antaki, S. Vehviläinen and I. Leudar (eds) *Conversation Analysis and Psychotherapy* (pp. 120–138), Cambridge: Cambridge University Press.

Virokannas, E. (2011) 'Identity categorization of motherhood in the context of drug abuse and child welfare services', *Qualitative Social Work*, 10(3): 329–345.

Volosinov, V.N. (1971) 'Reported speech', in L. Matejka and K. Promorska (eds) *Readings in Russian Poetics: Formalist and structuralist views* (pp. 149–175), Cambridge, MA: MIT Press.

Walsh, J. (2009) *Theories for Direct Social Work Practice*, Belmont, CA: Thomson, Brooks-Cole Publishing.

Wastell, D., White, S., Broadhurst, K., Peckover, S. and Pithouse, A. (2010) 'Children's services in the iron cage of performance management: street-level bureaucracy and the spectre of Švejkism', *International Journal of Social Welfare*, 19(3): 310–320.

Watson, D.R. (1990) 'Some features of the elicitation of confessions in murder interrogations', in G. Psathas (ed.) *Interaction Competence* (pp. 263–295), Lanham, MD: University Press of America.

Watson, J. (2011) 'Resistance is futile? Exploring the potential of motivational interviewing', *Journal of Social Work Practice*, 25(4): 465–479.

Webb, S. (2000) 'Some considerations of the validity of evidence-based practice in social work', *British Journal of Social Work*, 31(1): 57–79.

Weijts, W., Houtkoop, H. and Mullen, P. (1993) 'Talking delicacy: speaking about sexuality during gynaecological consultations', *Sociology of Health & Illness*, 15(3): 295–314.

Wells, K. (2010) 'A narrative analysis of one mother's story of child custody loss and regain', *Children and Youth Services Review*, 33(3): 439–447.

Wells, K. (2011) *Narrative Inquiry*, Oxford: Oxford University Press.

Wetherell, M. (2007) 'A step too far: discursive psychology, linguistic ethnography and questions of identity', *Journal of Sociolinguistics*, 11(5), 661–681.

Wetherell, M., Yates, S. and Taylor, S. (eds) (2001) *Discourse Theory and Practice: A reader*, London: Sage.

White, M. and Epston, D. (1990) *Narrative Means to Therapeutic Ends*, New York: W.W. Norton.

White, S. (2002) 'Accomplishing a case in paediatrics and child health: medicine and morality in inter-professional talk', *Sociology of Health and Illness*, 24(4): 409–35.

White, S., Hall, C. and Peckover, S. (2009) 'The descriptive tyranny of the common assessment framework: technologies of categorization and professional practice in child welfare', *British Journal of Social Work*, 39(7): 1197–1217.

White, S., Wastell, D., Broadhurst, K. and Hall, C. (2010) 'When policy o'erleaps itself: the "tragic tale" of the integrated children's system', *Critical Social Policy*, 30(3): 405–429.

Wikström, E. (2008) 'Boundary work as inner and outer dialogue: dieticians in Sweden', *Qualitative Research in Organizations and Management: An International Journal*, 3(1): 59–77.

Wilinska, M. and Henning, C. (2011) 'Old age identity in social welfare practice', *Qualitative Social Work*, 10(3): 346–363.

Wilks, T. (2005) 'Social work and narrative ethics', *British Journal of Social Work*, 35(6): 1249–1264.

Willig, C. (ed.) (1999) *Applied Discourse Analysis: Social and psychological interventions*, Buckingham: Open University Press.

Wittgenstein, L. (1953) *Philosophical Investigations*, New York: Macmillan.

Wood, L.A. and Kroger, R.O. (2000) *Doing Discourse Analysis: Method for analysing action in talk and text*, London: Sage.

Woods, A. (2011) 'Post-narrative: an appeal', *Narrative Inquiry*, 21(2): 399–406.

Wooffitt, R. (1992) *Telling Tales of the Unexpected: The organization of factual discourse*, Hemel Hempstead: Harvester Wheatsheaf.

Zimmerman, D.H. (1998) 'Identity, context and interaction', in C. Antaki and S. Widdicombe (eds) *Identities in Talk* (pp. 87–106), London: Sage.

AUTHOR INDEX

SUBJECT INDEX

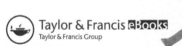